'Gillie Bolton holds the keys to healthier, happier, more robust living. In this delightful book, she unlocks doors, crates, and mystery chests of experience and emotion, expertly guiding us to our own hidden rooms, forgotten resources and undiscovered treasures.'

– *Kathleen Adams, Director, Center for Journal Therapy, USA*

'What a gift – Gillie Bolton's writing wisdom, creativity and humanity presented in a fresh and utterly accessible way. If you are interested in opening a door and crossing thresholds into creative adventure or personal discovery, here's a sensitive and learned guide. Bolton knows how writing can provide ways into and out of life's terrains, smooth or bumpy, shady or bright. With a light touch, she shares insights and learning. *The Writer's Key* offers practical writing exercises, mapped out carefully and enriched with reflections from other writers navigating diverse experience. For novices, this book will provide support with first steps. For the experienced, it's a re-energising reminder of how and why we write. For everyone, it's a clear message that we each have a key and, if we choose, we can take this author's ample encouragement to trust the process and "Write!"'

– *Fiona Hamilton, writer and Director of Orchard Foundation, UK*

'Gillie's book is an extraordinarily good read. Some of the keys are simple and easy to use, others are jewelled and more demanding to turn. It is a book which promotes the mysterious and irreducible, and is for times when spoken words aren't deep, wide or strong enough.'

– *Jeannie Wright, Director of Counselling and Psychotherapy Programmes, Warwick University, UK*

'Gillie Bolton has furnished a meeting and finding place for surprisingly new words and freshly understood old words. Reading this work of explorative exercises, observations, reflections and insights can make a difference. With *The Writer's Key* you can open hidden doors into your memories, dreams, and relations, unpack and repack your life stories. "Ask your writing!" she advises. Write your senses, chances and changes, sharing your expressive words with others.'

– *Juhani Ihanus, Professor of Psychology, University of Helsinki, Finland*

'*The Writer's Key* is an exciting and accessible way into creative writing for personal development; the many anecdotes and creative examples feed the reader, and the many ideas and imaginative exercises nourish the writer. This book shows the foundational ways in which writing can transform, release and motivate individuals as they travel through the sunlit and shadowed passages of life.'

– *Claire Williamson, Programme Leader, MSc in Creative Writing for Therapeutic Purposes, Metanoia Institute, London, UK*

'Gillie Bolton's *Writer's Key* is a supremely hopeful book, one that reveals in every page its author's belief in the resilience, wisdom and creativity of us all. In this book, the author opens up so many doors for us as readers, with her encouraging words and gentle tone, her expertise as a personal writing specialist, and the generous treasure trove of writing prompts and illustrations she provides.

Gillie Bolton brings years of personal and professional experience to fruition in this practical and inspirational guide to writing. Gently and with clarity and conviction, the author inspires us all to express our writer's voice, explore our unique selves, recognize our inner wisdom figures and realize the power we have to transform our lives.

The Writer's Key is a multi-faceted guide to writing for healing, meaning-making and enhanced self-development. In vivid, detailed ways, Bolton drives home the power of the writing process and inspires its readers to get out their favourite notebook and pen and proceed on their own creative journeys of discovery.'
– *Geri Chavis, Licensed Psychologist, Certified Poetry Therapist and Supervisor, USA*

'This book provides a gentle invitation to writing as a form of self-discovery, and quietly leads the user into some powerful moments of personal reflection. Highly recommended to anyone who is interested in learning more about the transformative potential of creative writing.'
– *John McLeod, Emeritus Professor of Counselling, Abertay University, Dundee, Scotland, and Adjunct Professor of Psychology, Oslo University, Norway*

'*The Writer's Key* is a necessary and inspirational book. It unlocks the secrets to the therapeutic potential of creative writing in all its forms. Gillie Bolton is a trustworthy, enthusiastic and invaluable guide for therapists and for those who know, instinctively, that writing may become a source of exploration, understanding and solace. Through her lucid chapters, examples and exercises, Gillie proves that there's no greater opportunity than that offered by a blank page and an itch to bring it alive with words.'
– *Robert Hamberger, poet, UK*

THE WRITER'S KEY

Writing for Therapy or Personal Development Series
Edited by Gillie Bolton

Writing for Therapy or Personal Development, a foundation library to a rapidly developing field, covers the theory and practice of key areas. Clearly exemplified, engaging and accessible, the series is appropriate for therapeutic, healthcare, or creative writing practitioners and facilitators, and for individual writers or courses.

other books in the series

Write Yourself
Creative Writing and Personal Development
Gillie Bolton
Foreword by Nicholas Mazza
ISBN 978 1 84905 110 1
eISBN 978 0 85700 308 9

Writing Works
A Resource Handbook for Therapeutic Writing Workshops and Activities
Edited by Gillie Bolton, Victoria Field and Kate Thompson
Foreword by Blake Morrison
ISBN 978 1 84310 468 1
eISBN 978 1 84642 549 3

Writing Routes
A Resource Handbook of Therapeutic Writing
Gillie Bolton, Victoria Field and Kate Thompson
Foreword by Gwyneth Lewis
ISBN 978 1 84905 107 1
eISBN 978 0 85700 303 4

Writing in Bereavement
A Creative Handbook
Jane Moss
ISBN 978 1 84905 212 2
eISBN 978 0 85700 450 5

Poetry and Story Therapy
The Healing Power of Creative Expression
Geri Giebel Chavis
ISBN 978 1 84905 832 2
eISBN 978 0 85700 311 9

THE
WRITER'S
KEY

Introducing Creative Solutions for Life

Gillie Bolton

Jessica Kingsley *Publishers*
London and Philadelphia

First published in 2014
by Jessica Kingsley Publishers
73 Collier Street
London N1 9BE, UK
and
400 Market Street, Suite 400
Philadelphia, PA 19106, USA

www.jkp.com

Copyright © Gillie Bolton 2014

Library of Congress Cataloging in Publication Data
Bolton, Gillie.
 The writer's key : creative solutions for life / Gillie Bolton.
   pages cm
 Includes bibliographical references.
 ISBN 978-1-84905-475-1 (alk. paper)
 1. Creative writing--Therapeutic use. 2. Self-care, Health. I. Title.
 RC489.W75B652 2014
 616.89'165--dc23
                    2013023986

British Library Cataloguing in Publication Data
A CIP catalogue record for this book is available from the British Library

ISBN 978 1 84905 475 1
eISBN 978 0 85700 854 1

Printed and bound in Great Britain by Bell and Bain Ltd, Glasgow

The Key is dedicated to Dan and Alice

CONTENTS

ACKNOWLEDGEMENTS

The Key has grown from a tiny seed, sown over 30 years ago, into a mighty tree in my life. This tree has sheltered many in its branches and roots; they in turn have nurtured the work, and I am greatly indebted. Like the mighty Ygdrassil of Nordic legend this tree's roots reach into hell where a dragon gnaws them, and its twigs touch angels.

I thank so many of my patients, students, mentees, supervisees, colleagues, friends, from the bottom of my heart for your openness and wisdom. You have given insight, allowed me to quote your writings, generously been willing for me to tell your stories. Many of you requested your name not to be put with your writing, some asked for first name only. Those who were happy for me to quote and name, I thank Inez de Beaufort, Jane Calne, Lizzie Chittleboro, Judy Clinton, Derek Collins, Francesca Creffield, Vicky Darling, Helena de Meza, Tom Heller, Helen Evans, Ruth Folit, Cecilia Forrestal, Fiona Friend, Nigel Gibbons, Carry Gorney, Caroline Hadley, Mark Halliday, Fiona Hamilton, Lucy Henshall, Seth Jenkinson, Karol Silovsky, John Latham, Caleb Lambert, Heidi Lyth, Erika Mansnerus, Sue McDonald, Angela McLean, Joan Michelson, Najwa Mounla, Eleanor Nesbitt, Dorothy Nimmo, Kathleen Russell, Rebecca Ship, Sue Sims, Helen Starkey, Monica Suswin, Sila Tarina, Jane Wilde, River Wolton, Yvonne Mak Yi Wood.

Robert Hamberger has hovered often, fertiliser and watering can in gentle hand. Kate Billingham in her forthright ever-loving way has wielded pruning knives. Michele Angelo Petrone pointed out unnoticed flowers and butterflies, before he joined the angels. Melanie Fein helped flowers bloom, and Sandy Sheehy and Julie Bittman polished fruit. My fellow critical poetry group *Off the Page* members picnicked in the shade with me: Rob Hamberger, John Latham, Joan Poulson, Andrew Rudd, Alicia Stubbersfield, Chris Woods.

Alice Rowland danced with me under this tree, and Dan Rowland chanted growth spells. Stephen Rowland helped me find the original tiny seed, cherished the fragile seedling, replanted it after storms and a hurricane, and always mulched, fed and watered: an ever-present presence.

PREFACE

I must unpack my heart with words.

HAMLET 2:2:594

Human lives are always storm-threatened; some of the storms are good, like getting a new job which can overturn a life completely with new places, faces, and new necessary ways of being. Many storms are caused by loss of job, loved one, health, or by clashes with colleague or partner. Garrison Keillor wrote of country children attending town schools in the cold north of America being paired with welcoming 'storm home' town-dwelling families for blizzard nights to keep them safe until it was safe to travel again (1985). We all need *storm homes* which offer a safe, free and accepting refuge at any time. And we need these *storm homes* also to offer us support in assessing, questioning, coming to terms with, understanding other points of view, and so on. This latter is just as vital, although much more challenging.

Hamlet said, 'I must unpack my heart with words.' In addition, in order to survive, develop despite adverse conditions, and make enduring and strong relationships, he could have done with *repacking* his heart with *new* or perhaps *freshly understood old* words.

Writing can help us find these words, can give us this strong refuge and power to listen to ourselves critically in order to reshape our lives. *The Writer's Key*, as its name suggests, offers a way of unlocking the door.

Writing is effective partly because it is undertaken in the safety of solitude and silence; the white page itself is a form of silence; a silent frame for these important yet private words. It can be completely safely private until we choose to share it with a carefully chosen other. The stories we write are tentative, half formulated, not yet fully known to us, because this writing is explorative and expressive rather than previously thought out. And we can feel confident to create it in this otherwise exposing way because nobody knows yet what these words are which land on the white page. We use writing, rather than talking, to enable the exploration, the *unpacking* and *repacking of words*.

What we write each time is 'a version, but never a final one'. *Key* writing is never final, so we can continue to write, rewrite, question, reassess. Our muddle gradually becomes clearer; sometimes to such an extent that things can seem to become entirely different from how we had always thought they were, or assumed them to be. Writing enables us to take stock of assumptions and taken-for-granteds, sometimes even to chuck them all out and find stronger life foundations.

As a young woman I found this *Key* quite by chance, at a time when my life had become impossible due to a legacy of childhood abuse. Using writing to unpack and repack my heart, mind and spirit was demanding; I accepted no half measures. I then devoted the rest of my life's research and practice to developing writing as an effective way to reflect upon and develop both work and personal life. My practice and research has principally been with medical and other helping professionals, and with hospice and other terminally ill patients including children. Through all this, I have continued to write and use writing to understand things about my self, work, children, grandchildren, and the ongoing repercussions from my early abuse. *The Writer's Key* is the culmination of this career which has included publication of many books, academic papers and other materials for professionals.

The author and novelist Jeanette Winterson published a memoir about how she did much more than survive her own childhood abuse. Literature was an early *storm home* and source of insight; later she discovered how writing could enable her to *pack and repack her heart*. Here is her reflection upon silence:

> There are so many things that we can't say because they are so painful… When we tell a story we exercise control, but in such a way as to leave a gap, an opening. It is a version, but never a final one. And perhaps we hope that the silences will be heard by someone else, and the story can continue, be retold. When we write we offer the silence as much as the story. Words are part of silence that can be spoken. (Winterson 2011, p.8)

The Writer's Key suggests many different ways to write, to discover and understand more about ourselves and those near us, and to see more in life. This writing is imaginative and illuminative, an enjoyable straightforward way to explore little-known and under-appreciated parts of ourselves, our lives and environments. No teacher or boss waits, red pen poised, to criticise: our writing belongs to us. These creative ways of writing are dynamic: full of possibilities for those who have been writing for years, as well as those completely new to it. These methods prevent getting bogged down and repetitive, or stuck in negative memories and thoughts. They open storehouses of information, advice, inspirations, explanations and examples. People exclaim, 'I can't believe I've written that', 'Is this my writing?', 'It only took fifteen minutes!'

HOW TO USE THE WRITER'S KEY

The Writer's Key is practical and informative, with suggestions, advice, strategies and examples from people in a very wide range of situations. Reading it straight through could be a good beginning. An alternative would be to go to the parts which seem appropriate at the time. The chapters are ordered in a way I think is developmental. Every reader and writer is different, however, and the chapters can well be read in different orders. Whatever order it's read in, reading the first three chapters before any of the others will be beneficial. The suggested ways of writing in these chapters are foundational, particularly what I call the *Six Minute Write*, which is an initial explorative and expressive splurge laying the ground each writing session for further writing.

Each chapter ends with *Write!*, a menu of writing suggestions and strategies. All the major exercises in *The Writer's Key* are listed in the appendices, whether from within chapters, or from the *Write!* sections at the end. They are sorted in two ways: in Appendix A they are listed accordingly to type of writing activity (e.g. poetry); in Appendix B they are listed according to the area of life they can help with (e.g. depression). Some suggestions may be preferred to others: people are different and write in different ways. Try! Play around with the suggestions, altering them according to need and want. Stop halfway through an exercise if it feels boring or too frustrating, or even painful; it may engross another time. Another idea might demand to be returned to time and time again. Writing's like that. Take it lightly, follow its lead. A new personal writer said, 'If I'm stuck I know now to find different, more imaginative ways to start. I previously found writing always in the same way just reinforced and fixed obsessive thoughts.'

The Writer's Key arises from my own practice, and people I have worked with over many years. Every writing suggestion has been used by one or more; many have generously given permission for their writing to be quoted as examples.

Writing is the silver lining in the dark cloud of my mental illness and quite honestly the only thing that makes my life bearable, even joyful, like a rose in winter, like a day-trip to the lighter side of the moon, like a favourite chair in a cold room.

Tom

Writing even got me to see that failing the all important job interview was, perhaps, even a blessing in disguise and led me to rethink my priorities. And I got the next job, and it was far better both for me and for my family!

Leroy

Sometimes we don't even understand how the writing has helped, but yet know that it certainly has:

Deinacrida elegans
distinctively detailed
delicately endangered
In the high country cracks of my mind

Fractured, fissured, windswept and dry
but not barren;
Tangled matagouri
proof of life

This poem is about an endangered native gecko (lizard) that lives in the dry hills of an area in New Zealand South Island high country. The matagouri plant a twisted, rough and thorny native, that seems to thrive in this landscape. Really it's a statement of how I was feeling in myself at the end of my PhD – an inhospitable ground for fertile thoughts, a fragile existence! Writing remains a difficult task. The fact that we are still dealing with ongoing sequelae from the (Christchurch) earthquakes is mixed up with my feelings about writing, in a way that I can't explain properly.

Angela McLean

I hope my words reach out to help wings on your pen sprout and grow. I hope they help you stop fearing the destructive instructional red pen. Whoever you are, whatever your work, way of life, beliefs, hobbies, your written words may be the key to bring you closer to your dreams, memories, your world and the people in it.

CHAPTER 1

The Writer's Key

An Introduction

Our lives are ours. Our dreams, ambitions, joys, successes, inspirations and memories belong to us, as do our fears, anxieties, sorrows and pain. All these are ours to make the best of we can. Held, or wielded well, they are our riches. The key is in our own hands.

When life becomes difficult or even out of hand due to illness, loss or work problems, the wisest person to turn to is often oneself. Personal writing's artistic power to give insight has been unrecognised next to more glamorous cousins, art, music, drama, dance. Now in our age of complexity, the simplicity of pushing a pen or pencil over a page has come into its own. People want to express themselves, explore what is inside them, experiment with different ways of knowing, perceiving and being. *The Writer's Key* unlocks secrets of how to do this.

Awareness of life, in all its varied aspects, can be likened to a set of keys. Imagine a home where some rooms and parts of the garden are open, full of soft light and natural shade, and some closed or even locked. Some keys are lost or even thrown away. Battering down doors will disturb the peace. Pretending these locked places aren't there doesn't work: trying to forget something makes us remember it in increasingly damaging ways.

Writing can help find the keys, enabling much more of the building to be used for living and working. It can help re-find boarded-up doors, uncover locks, winkle dust out of keyholes, oil rusted-up mechanisms, turn keys, and push hard against the stuff which has collected over time, holding the door closed.

Writing can help find windows in gloomy parts of life, help throw shutters open to let in light and air. Our minds' secret gardens have old roses needing pruning, weeding, fertilising. Grass can be mown, brambles and briars rooted out and cut away to enable rare bulbs to flower.

A word meaning hostage
Imprisons my fancies.
Each syllable pins
That gorgeous blue butterfly
Inside a paragraph.

If I were a writer
I'd make you fly
or cry of love.
I'd feed you to a whale.
Realising yourself
You wouldn't notice me
at all.

Helena de Meza

A man was terrified of flying. When he realised promotion meant foreign business trips he took time and space to write everything he could think of about flying. He began crying uncontrollably, recalling returning from a family holiday. His father had had a heart attack abroad and bringing him in the aeroplane to die at home had been a nightmare. Writing helped him realise he'd transferred his memory of horror onto the flight rather than the incident. He talked to his brother and mother; they reminisced and cried together. He subsequently gained promotion and discovered a joy in foreign places, though latterly he began to seek railway or sea alternatives to use less carbon.

The Key offers writers' methods for gaining initial inspirations: anyone who can put words on a page can do it. We are all artists to some extent. Though there is no need for us to craft this writing into publishable novels, poems, plays (though of course this is always possible, with time and patience).

Creative expression can open up pathways to a full range of aspects of our selves. Our culture has so privileged logical approaches that creative ways of thinking have either become downgraded as not useful or considered only the province of special people: artists. At the tenth-century Japanese court everyone had to write tiny stylised poems about beauty: in that culture these artistic abilities were exalted above the rational and logical.

Creativity can be playful. Art can take us back to the kind of exploring we left behind with our childhoods (in words, paint, clay, movement). In creative exploration, we aren't anxious about getting it right (because there isn't a right) or afraid of appearing foolish or wrong. This confidence in uncertainty is possible because we know we need share things with others only when we are ready. Musicians *play* instruments, sometimes alone so no-one hears their mistakes and experiments: *Key* writing plays words in private. This can give us the confidence we need.

> Then…almost by magic, I was aware of a little voice. A quietly spoken soothing voice, just telling me to do what came naturally. That I am OK, and I don't have to follow instructions if I don't want to, and why don't I write about IT? IT being the fear, and what was happening to me right there and then. So I picked up my pen and told myself to just write whatever came, and that it would be OK whatever appeared. Relief! The anxious feelings began to subside. I turned off the instructions on the screen, and tuned in to myself and discovered, once more, the guidance I needed… The person I seek is right here, holding this pen. The container is my journal. As I write I tap into the richest wisdom of the universe.
>
> *Sue McDonald*

Our lives are a kaleidoscope of influences, events, people, places, long periods of uneventful work and domesticity varied by bursts of drama. From the perspective of the future, or from space, my life's pattern would be apparent, but from its lived centre it can feel out of control and incomprehensible. It can be too easy to focus on minor elements and miss the big one, or not grasp opportunities.

Life wobbles us off balance now and then: instabilities with colleagues, work issues, family, health, housing are unavoidable. Sometimes we know exactly what has gone wrong, and what to do about it; too often we don't. Sometimes we try to live with anxiety and lowness of spirits. Writing can give inspiration for viewing and dealing with things more positively and creatively. A medieval monk in Durham wrote, 'the writing desk is tranquillity of the heart'. More recently an ex-coal-miner wrote:

> After being made compulsorily redundant I started night school as I couldn't spell. I found out I am dyslexic. Once I knew the problems I could turn them to my advantage. Writing was once a dread but now it's a joy. I can get all my fears, hates and anger out of my mind and onto the paper.

The Writer's Key gives positive ways to look at and explore life, strategies which can create unexpected understanding and awareness. Stress can so readily pull us down and narrow our view. Writing can draw on elements from our whole being and life situation, rather than focusing directly on problems, anxieties or loss. Positive aspects can come clearly into view because they are more powerful than negative, however hard this is to believe at times. Energy and hopefulness with which to tackle difficulties or despair, and awareness of width and depth rather than the narrowly painful, can come into view. Exhilarating at times, as we never know what might appear on the page, writing can foster greater awareness of joy and pleasure, and put horrors or dullness into deeper and wider perspective, helping us see life's picture in fuller colour and light. It can also bring tears along the way, but healing tears of understanding.

Writing can bring heavy thoughts and memories to the surface, which can be uncomfortable or even difficult at the time. Facing painful issues through the helpful medium of writing can ultimately lighten them, however, if they are tackled positively, and good self-enhancing memories also recalled. *The Writer's Key* gives positive strategies to prevent writing becoming depressing or even frightening.

Finding the Keys

Once upon a time a student set off to search for the truth. On advice from elders, our seeker travelled long and arduous weeks by boat, horse, ox wagon, but mostly on foot, eventually to arrive at a refuge high in misty mountains. There the wisest person on earth dwelt, or so had been promised. Our seeker after the truth patiently entered the ways of the place, eating humble food, sweeping floors, and meditating daily. The meditation was never for a set time, however, which became increasingly frustrating: some days the bell was rung after an hour, sometimes six minutes, once after six hours. The student became more and more irritated, particularly as there never seemed any possibility of a tutorial with the wise one.

Eventually, in a fit of anger at the waste of youth, our seeker got up, strode towards the huge yet gentle sounding bell, seized the beater and struck it hard. Sitting down in fear and trembling at such audacity, the student was amazed to see the wise one get up slowly, shuffle forwards, bow deeply and say 'You have grasped the key to the important lesson in wisdom.'

I retell this ancient story because the student discovers her or his own power. He or she learns that wisdom is within our own grasp: it cannot be given by another, however wise. We must all ring our own bells, and never give others authority to ring them for us. The mysteriously beautiful high place soon becomes home to the student, who learns fascinatedly and fast from then onwards.

Expressive, explorative personal writing helps develop that wisdom. And – although it's hard to believe before starting – it's straightforward and enjoyable. Basic writing equipment, and skills to write a list or letter are all that are needed. We also need trust it'll work for us, respect for ourselves and our strength and ability to do it, and enough self-care to gift ourselves a few minutes every day or every now and then: just for me and nobody else. Fiona Hamilton said of her work, 'Holding [writing] sessions in a prison afforded a prisoner the chance to hear "What you've done is really good" for the first time in his life.'

WHAT IS CREATIVITY?

Once the creative self comes from behind the locked door and wields pen or pencil: that's when writing begins.

Other writers have put this in different ways. French philosopher Hélène Cixous said she raided her jewellery box for its wealth; writing gave her the key she needed. Poet Seamus Heaney digs with his pen like a spade in peat. He also likened writing to letting a bucket down a well-shaft, keeping trying until the bucket fills with enticing water. The novelist Virginia Woolf described herself as fishing: 'letting her imagination sweep unchecked round every rock and cranny of the world that lies submerged in the depths of our unconscious being' (Woolf 1979[1931], p.60). Poet Ted Hughes had to 'outwit his own inner police system' (Hughes 1982, p.7).

Key writing methods can enable creative observations, ideas, thoughts and reflections. Rational logical thought can tend to keep the jewellery box locked, the pen just a pen not a spade, and the bucket swinging up empty of life-giving spring-water. The ancient philosopher Plato called writing the *crutch of memory*. Writers lean on it, let it help them go much further than without. Eleanor was struggling with cancer when she wrote this:

Even in the dark, one sleepless night, I wrote blindly, capturing images and fleeting thoughts without the fear that they would have evaporated by the morning. I would rather throw them away in the cold light of day than feel that I had let something precious and fleeting slip past irretrievably. Both writing and reading my diary entries have clarified my feelings and ideas.

Eleanor Nesbitt (1996/1997, pp.7–9)

What we want and need to write is there inside us: different approaches are ways of allowing us to attend to it properly. There must be as many strategies as there are occasions when people write. Ted Hughes said 'writers have invented all kinds of games to get past their own censorship' (Hughes 1982, p.7). These games help find the right earth to dig with the right spade; find the right depth in the well; lull the policeman to sleep; unlock the jewellery box.

Often we feel as if there's nothing at all there to write, yet this is precisely the place to start. A bored nothing-seeming mind is a crucible of creativity: a state of mind seeking something definite to grapple with. Given space, respect, trust and perseverance, the key will turn so the door slips open.

Some writing will be dynamic and exciting, leading further; some will inevitably seem mere scribble. Scientists spend years testing slight variations on hypotheses before discovering life-changing formulae. Sometimes it feels as though I'm biting to life's core when I write, sometimes I can't even get my teeth through the skin. There's nothing clever, mystical or magical about it, however, nothing which is the special province of people born with artistic powers. It just uses our ordinary everyday words: grasp them.

Many people when they start are inevitably hesitant and uncertain. Creativity takes us into the unknown, into areas where we are uncertain of ourselves and what we know, feel, remember. Writing in *Key* ways can take courage to step over the boundaries of certainty into the great unexplored Land of Uncertainty. The more I put into something, the more I receive. Chris Woods is a family medical practitioner and poet; he writes:

From a doctor's perspective I found the act of writing allows exploration of the thoughts and feelings of my patients, the world around me and myself. Exploration brings understanding. It allows me to imaginatively enter into the experiences of my patients and to try and understand their problems. With understanding hopefully comes wisdom and ability to treat effectively. The act of writing can be therapeutic to patients and doctors alike.

In depression, the channelling of that dark energy through the creative process can be healing in its own right. I have often asked patients simply to write down what they are thinking and feeling. The very act of writing is often therapeutic and a release. It allows patients to explore and eventually understand their problems. Effective treatment and healing can follow. Doctors and patients can take this further if they wish and continue along the path of self-discovery.

First Thing
He wakes early
and pushes back blankets
before night covers him again.

He stumbles along
to the bathroom,
tries to wash the shadows away.

Downstairs, in the silence
before the house wakes,
he sits down,

turns on the lamp
and feels safe
within its tent of light.

He begins to write
and black ink is shadow
released across the page.

Chris Woods (2008, p.31)

WHAT DO YOU WANT?

'Writing can't change a criminal into an innocent person!' a lawyer once snapped at me. Of course it can't. But it can make a tremendous difference to their understanding of the role of the crime in their lives. And writing letters to, and receiving them from, their victim can deepen this awareness. Writing can also support lawyers themselves towards greater clarity about the human situations, and possible motives of their clients.

Writing cannot mend physical disease or injury either, but it can be very helpful. Human bodies, minds and spirits are bonded together, making whole integrated people: state of mind and spirit affects the body. Contented people don't tend to get so ill, they experience less severe symptoms when they do, are able to cope with severe symptoms better and recover more quickly. And what makes us happier? Not being terrified of what's going on inside. Being able to ask for what we want. Accepting as far as we can where we are in life.

Often people want but don't know what. Writing to discover vital wants and needs can help prevent reaching for the moon. Living with *if only…* can be draining and bullying.

> …the 'if only'
> sentences circle and circle like a hawk going for the kill
> with the speed of iron filings attracted to a magnetic pole
> like lemmings marching over that cliff top…
>
> *Monica*

My three-year-old granddaughter recently asked her grandfather to bring his longest ladder to fetch her the moon; she later told me her baby sister wanted the sky. We all have the right to want. We are born and die wanting: and that's OK. What isn't OK is constantly trying not to want, believing it's wrong. This leads to living with constant frustration, and perhaps jealousy of those who seem to have.

Wanting is so often associated with guilt, once we are older than three. Listening to ourselves coherently, lovingly, and without guilt, can enable us to understand and communicate with the wanting self, as well as the loving and wise. We are the greatest authority on ourselves, yet we are extraordinarily deaf to the 'still small voices' inside which lighten understanding. Gaining insight can help towards possible wants, and acceptance of the impossibility of others. Here is Caleb Lambert's journal wish list, when he was very ill:

I wish

- I hadn't got ill

- I could stop feeling sick (though I've managed to write this without interruption)

- I may make a full recovery

- I may find a new direction/new possibilities in my work

- That my mum will die peacefully and without pain

- That A- may maintain her health and recovery

- I could be less grumpy (not hard! That one's definitely within my control!)

Is that it? No other things are immediately springing to mind. It doesn't seem a very long list. But maybe being ill helps you focus on priorities, what really counts…

Caleb Lambert

Art creates something which wasn't there before, and everyone feels better when they make something. People often enter a room hesitantly for a creative or reflective writing workshop. They think and feel, 'I can't write; what AM I doing here?' They would turn and run if they weren't too grown-up. Within an hour beaming faces fill the room, still sensitive and tentative, but certain now they can create new things which they and others find interesting and even thrilling.

WHY WRITING?

Why writing rather than talking or thinking? Writing is qualitatively different from either. Here is a compilation from many writers saying why they write.

Why I write
I write to entertain
To find out what I feel
I begin to like myself more
I enjoy the mental challenge
It gives me a sense of freedom
There's a sense of power in creation
I write because others do: we can share together
I need to tell stories, create poems, narratives, fables
A finished piece gives immense satisfaction and achievement

I gain insight into who I am, what I want and how I want to live my
life

It brings me order and something positive, from confusion and
negativity

I don't dump the pain as in therapy: it remains mine and is lessened
creatively

I learn where my feelings are coming from, what they connect to, so I
can leave them behind, look beyond them

Novelist and journalist Blake Morrison said, 'writing a book about my
father [*And When Did You Last See Your Father?*] enabled me to move from
not being able to speak of him coherently during the year after his death to
being able to' (2005, p.1).

The Key way of writing:

1. is a creative way of discovering what we think, feel, know, understand,
    remember, hope, fear, are joyful or stressed or anxious about. It helps
    closer observation: hearing, seeing, smelling, tasting, feeling in a
    new way. And keen observation can enable insight.

2. is a fluid and open way of thinking aloud on the page; as such
    it cannot be got wrong. I can experiment with crazy ideas,
    fictionalised memories and wild possible solutions to problems, in as
    ungrammatical, misspelt disordered way as I like. Such explorations,
    whatever they are, are always of value to me. If I want to rethink
    any, redraft for someone else to read, I can do that, and that'll be
    right too.

3. is a perfect listener: it will not recoil in horror, gasp in amazement,
    laugh embarrassingly or embarrassedly, or make any other response.
    I communicate with myself as first reader. Even if someone else
    might read it later, I reread first, choosing the words I wish to
    communicate. This is so different from talking: a listener cannot be
    asked to un-hear what they've been told.

4. belongs to its writer: it's not for publication, nor as an explanation to
    anyone else, not even for communication with nearest and dearest.
    Though sharing writing with one or two people can be useful at a
    later stage.

5. is endlessly patient of changes of mind. It can be rewritten as many times as wished, or stopped, or put away unread, rubbed out, deleted, ripped up, flushed away, burned even. It will never remonstrate: 'but yesterday you said…'

6. helps me get quickly to the point of what I need to reflect on or communicate. As I am my own first reader, there's no point in waffling: I don't need to explain or cover myself. Writing is slower and harder on the hand than talking, so I might as well get to the point quickly.

7. will not fade, like memory. It never forgets or muddles what's been said. Faithful and silent it keeps my words in trust until I decide to share them, or not.

8. can prevent thoughts from circling round and round the mind fruitlessly. Putting them down on the page can distance them: still to be thought about but in a kinder, less spiralling manner.

9. can be available at any appropriate time or place. Human listeners are often too busy, get bored of hearing about the same thing time and again, or are expensive (if therapists).

10. can help sort things out in my head before sharing them with others: useful at work or other relationships where care is needed. Thoughts and feelings (such as anger) can be practised and redrafted before being shared with the significant other. When the worst of it (if it is anger) has been yelled onto the paper, what I really want or need to communicate will be clarified.

11. can help communication with others. Sharing a key piece of reflective writing with someone I need to talk to can speed the beginning of a conversation.

12. encourages experimentation, playing with images. Images, particularly metaphor, can be keys to understanding (see Chapter 7).

13. enables formatively playful involvement in argument and debate. Contradictory ideas, theories and opposing arguments can be tried out, until thinking is clarified.

The simple action of putting words on a page can begin to help us find out what we think, believe and know; and to understand and value our possession of greatest value: ordinary everyday life and work. A challenge is allowing myself to be open to whatever writing might happen onto the paper, without censoring it.

Life's priorities often seem unclear: we worry about all sorts of things. People with life-threatening diseases like cancer often know there are only a few really important things to worry about in life, and do not waste precious time and energy with anxiety about work or the many myriad things others ruin their life with. We can borrow some of their certainty without their tragedy. They know the greatest prizes on earth are health of loved ones and oneself, and the ability to enjoy our beautiful world with justice, trust, respect, care, regard for others, honesty, joy. Michele was a painter struggling with cancer; waking after a dream he wrote this:

> I know who the tattooed intruder is. He is my cancer. He has no name. Only a description. Yet he is a part of me I don't recognise. That is what brings tears to my eyes. In the calm darkness. In the stillness of the night emerges death. I want to think it is only a shadow, a sign, a symbol, a possibility. Not a fact this time. But it is a possibility I am aware of. A possibility I want to deny. Another throat cracked, teeth clenched, sick stomach, body shuddering tear swells in my eyes. Blurring my vision…

> I'm reminded of an Antoine de Saint-Exupéry quote that the beauty of the desert is that it conceals a well. Oh where is that well?

> …

> *It was cathartic to write this. I wrote as if recalling a dream/nightmare literally on the ward at 4am, just after waking and it helped me gather my feelings and emotions, my fears and my concerns, where I was and how I was. It is really hard to be able to express your feelings in the hospital environment and even though the dream was startling, frightening, it helped me place myself, express myself to myself and that was such a release.*

> *The truth is – it is frightening. It was also hard to write it up. But it was the eye of the storm and I was able to take issues on board. And then it became the basis of questions, that I probably wouldn't have asked my consultant about, and that gave me in turn more answers that has given me more confidence about the treatment. Funny how these things work.*
> *Michele Angelo Petrone (2002, p.30)*

Why writing is personally and professionally beneficial is clear. Now we turn to the treasure chest of how to begin writing.

WRITE!

1. Find a time and place where you can be alone with your writing for at least 20 minutes, where you feel relaxed and comfortable.

2. Write without thinking about commas and full stops, correct spelling, or proper form. Much of this writing will feel like the middle of something, since middles are where most things happen. You might fear it's a muddle; writings like this – done with no previous thinking – are often perfectly formed, however, and easy to understand. Grammar, spelling and sorting out a beginning, middle and end can be dealt with later if you wish to share it with another.

3. We assume we know so much about ourselves; writing down these assumptions can be enlightening. Here are sentence beginnings for you to continue from, writing a lot or a little: just whatever seems right to you. Allow your hand to do the thinking: put the pen on the page and see what comes. No-one else will read this unless you expressly wish them to. Try one or two now, and return every now and then to write from another one. Writing from the same one on different occasions can be illuminating: you do know a huge variety of stuff which this can bring to light.

   - I am…

   - I know…

   - I think…

   - I believe…

   - I remember…

   - I feel…

   - I want…

   - I wish…

   - I can…

- I wonder…

- I hope…

- I was told…

- I promise myself I will…

You'll notice that none begin with 'I should…', 'I ought…', 'I must…' This writing is about being positive and genuinely enquiring; it's the only way to find out the useful, interesting things. *Should* and *ought* and their ilk cause locks to jam, keys to rust, easing oil to turn to water, and door-handles to snap.

4. Write the story of your life, or perhaps just your work, or love, or artistic, life.

   a. Start wherever you like. Write as much or as little as you like, and for as long, about different elements. You might find you've written your entire life story in two pages. Or perhaps after 20 minutes you are still describing your birth and first years. That's OK; it doesn't matter if you never write any more. Or you could carry on another time.

   b. Give your life story a title, as if it were a film.

5. Read through your writing to yourself to see what you've written. Add or alter it in any way you like. Pay no attention to grammar, spelling and proper form at this stage unless you really want to; otherwise leave it as notes. Share it with someone else if you wish, or just keep it in your notebook.

CHAPTER 2

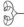

Beginning

Significant change and development is often unexpected, and sometimes even startling. How do some people open previously unperceived doors and have the courage to step through into new and challenging worlds? They open their minds to any possibility, however unlikely seeming; they willingly allow themselves not to know, and to stay with that not knowing until a dynamic possibility arrives. Some use writing as an enabling strategy. This writing has by its nature to be unplanned and explorative. Art takes the artist, or would-be-artist, by the hand and leads them, rather than the artist deciding what they want to do, making a plan and sticking to it; writing is no different. It can take courage to accept such a challenge. This chapter offers a foundation creative method which can be used to start every writing session. When and where to write can also be significant and will also be addressed, as will with whom to share writing, and when.

Why writing rather than talking to a friend? This writing uses different parts of us than talking to another. It is private: no-one will listen or read unless specifically invited. So the hand can be invited to think straight onto the page, potentially taking us more directly to our most vital issues. Like a game of football, where the players obey rules but no-one knows where the ball will go, nor who might make a brilliant catch or goal, this is very different from ordered planned essay or report. Such writing allows ideas, thoughts, feelings, memories, inspirations to tumble onto the page relatively unchecked. It can then be read to find out what what's there, or put away unread in a locked drawer for a later day, or redrafted to be shared with another, or even burned not read at all.

BASICS

Where and when we write can really affect the pace and flow of writing, and even what is written. Creativity is affected by so many things, some of them seemingly tiny. Some people write well in the morning but not the afternoon, some better in summer than winter. Some have bursts for weeks and then nothing (that's me); sometimes the computer might be good to write on, sometimes very much not, and a pencil is needed. Some respond well to making a clear plan and sticking to it as far as possible; to others this would spell death to their creativity.

An initial go at writing sometimes doesn't feel good, so it's worth trying a different place and/or time, and/or different materials. Pencil and paper create different results to computers; black fountain pen on thick new paper different from blue biro on second-hand scraps, and different again from a thick red felt-tip on flip-chart paper. Writing in the middle of the night, early morning hours, by the sea or a river, in a café or library, on a hilltop, or in bed – can make it different too. This writing is ours to experiment with.

I write in all sorts of places and at all sorts of times. In bed on waking in the morning when I'm alone; in the middle of the night within the glowing circle of a lamp; on top of the moor (I live in England's Peak District); by a river: green-bordered Derwent with its wagtails and water-rats, London's Thames, or the Cam at Cambridge's Grantchester Meadows with willows and punts. A few strangers at a distance is OK, but I don't like anyone other than my husband nearby (he never asks questions, knowing I'll talk when the time's right). Train journeys with their sense of boundedness are great. My all-time favourite is sprawled on the hearthrug with my husband playing Schubert on the piano. Here, a poet discovers where she could write.

Rarely have words forsaken me. Or it seems that the shock of my husband's sudden death stopped words as nothing before. This was in stark contrast to the death of my mother which I shared in its unremitting approach in long hours seated at her bedside. Around her dying days, I wrote a whole note-book. For solace I told myself my mother was 'full of years'. But the death of my life-mate was the death of a life I had not imagined coming to an end. It was a mild December day when without warning, my husband died on his way to work. Six months later I found I had scribbled something that night, a scrawl on a torn notebook page. This jolted me because my memory was of a shock so deep, I had been rendered mute.

Then it was summer. By fluke and luck I was able to escape to the American mid-west. I was afraid that I wouldn't be able to write at all;

that, freed from home, I would be pulled into grief as into a closed closet. But just the opposite. Later I would realise that the separation from home allowed me to work on this material and that inside our home, with the ordinary as memorials, I faced a struggle of a different order. In my own home it proved difficult if not impossible to transform my loss into writing.

Joan Michelson

SIX MINUTE WRITING: THE FOUNDATION

Going on an adventure by putting one foot in front of the other and seeing where it led is how Bilbo Baggins, J.R.R. Tolkein's character, described his life-changing experience. We can do the same with words. In this most basic writing method, the *Six Minute Write,* words determine where they want to go. Reading them afterwards, I find out what they've said. This follow-the-flow-of-my-mind, key to all writing, is the secret of much poetry, fiction, playwriting, autobiography, journal writing.

For this writing we invent our own rules. My writing is mine to do what I want with. Nobody else is going to see it unless I decide they may, so it's OK if it only makes sense to me. If I want someone else to read it, I can redraft it later with correct full stops, paragraphs, spelling, verbs, handwriting, and proper ways of beginning and ending. And I can cut out or alter bits I'd rather another reader didn't see. This is how I start:

- Take whatever materials feel good for today; this might be very different one time from another.

- Choose where to sit: under a tree, at the kitchen table, somewhere miles from home or office.

- Choose a peaceful time with at least 20 minutes UNINTERRUPTED, and ALONE.

- Settle comfortably.

- Allow the writing to write itself for at least six minutes WITHOUT STOPPING, without rereading, and as far as possible without thinking about it. Try not to sit and think AT ALL before beginning: put the pen or pencil on the paper and start writing, in mid-sentence if necessary: allow the hand on the paper to do the initial thinking.

- Our minds hop around, so well might this writing. Allow it to fall onto the paper: descriptions; shopping lists, moans about traffic, weather, children, colleagues; an account of something that happened; last night's dream; work or dinner plans: it doesn't matter what it is. Don't stop to question anything: write without thinking.

- We don't think in sentences or logical sequences, so neither might this writing. Only include punctuation, correct grammar and spelling which occurs naturally. Write FOLLOWING the FLOW for six minutes.

- If it gets stuck, just rewrite the last sentence, or look up and describe the surroundings.

- Whatever we write will be right for now; we might want to change things later, perhaps remembering things better or having rethought them. Or the spelling, punctuation and grammar might be far from perfect. None of these things matter for now; what matters is getting the gist of what I think, feel, know, remember, wonder, believe down now. With this kind of open approach it's impossible to think of such explorative expression as wrong.

Why SIX minutes flow-of-the-mind writing? I can't remember, as I began many years ago. Five was too short and seven not right somehow. Six minutes is one tenth of an hour, and ten the natural human numerical base (the word digit means both number and finger or toe). Three more lots of six minutes would be a 24 minute write: a good normal concentration length.

It is key of keys to the mansion of creative expressive and explorative writing. After a *Six Minute Write*, a woman realised she had to change her job. Acting on it immediately she shortly gained a distinguished CEO role. Every writer finds, however, that although sometimes this writing is an adventure, at other times it never even puts its hand on the door to go out. And sometimes we know what we want to write before beginning and at other times really don't. One of the secrets of writing is to keep doing it even when there seems to be nothing there, because:

1. writing, just as life, offers a muddle of the good, the bad and the boring: it might seem dull one minute, and full of vitality and significance the next

2. things hold different meanings at different times: a piece of writing might seem irrelevant or nondescript one day: but prove insightful later.

We write *six minutes* to clear the mind, to set the scene, to unburden from the trivia of life, and find a way through to the real 'stuff' that is within us all. I remember vividly thinking when I first wrote 'What does she mean *just write*?'

Six minutes – not long you think – but oh how much ground can be covered when you just let the pen do the work. Each time something special seems to happen and a thread of a story or a long forgotten experience pops back into sharp focus like a jack-in-the-box opening up to reveal itself.

Suddenly there it is, the *stuff* for the next writing, and we got there in only six minutes, not after hours of worrying or pondering what to do and how.

The sound of silence, the clearing of heads, the blank page waiting eagerly with the uncluttered freshness of a new day ahead – its content as yet unknown. The burdens of a busy mind shaken off, and the writing ahead waiting to unfold in front of our eyes like a water lily opening in the summer sunshine to reveal its inner beauty.

Lucy Henshall

SHARING WRITING

Personal writing can be completely private and never read by another; writing, however brilliant, does not need to be public in any way. Or certain pieces can, on careful reading and reflection, be selected to read to, or be read by, a trusted other; or it can be redrafted first, unsharable bits taken out or altered perhaps.

Finding the right person to share with – carefully, confidentially and trustingly – adds to the benefit of this writing: 'a good listener empowers the writing'. One personal writer I know reads closely, redrafts sometimes more sometimes less, then types out passages she wishes to read to her carefully chosen first reader: 'your honest receiving makes the writing even more real'. It's worth selecting the other reader carefully; they might be colleague, life partner, parent, best friend, or therapist, doctor or life-coach, or perhaps a creative writing partner, or writers' group.

And it's worth taking care about when to share. The other will read much better if in a receptive mood, not thinking about something else, or too tired. They might rather read it silently to themselves, or aloud, or have it read to them, whichever seems appropriate. And it can be done differently at different times.

My personal writing is never read by anyone, and only very rarely do I read a passage to my husband. Though I do redraft certain bits as poems.

FURTHER WRITING

Writing often has its own momentum, pushing ahead for far longer than six minutes. Sometimes the *Six Minute Write* offers inspirations for further writing, as Lucy points out above.

Giving the hand permission to write whatever comes with minimal thought about content or rules can facilitate beginning, as it does away with that scary thing, a blank sheet of paper. It can also turn up inspirations, or list and settle dominating day-to-day concerns which need to be put on one side. Further writing will clearly need some thought about content, but the pen or pencil can take the lead with little awareness of rules of grammar, form and structure. These have their place, but later.

Exploring personal experience can open up the next stage of writing. We know our own life and experience best. Sila wrote about trying to stop taking heroin.

> If taking opium is like stepping off a moving train, smoking crack is flying off it. Leaving the train in pieces. Day of tears and fears. Fragility. A trembling inside as if something died. Felt something again as if melting ice burned in my eyes down hot cheeks. Ice like fire.

> That silent part of me I am afraid of that I keep protected can no longer stay in its shell. Some might call it a soul or the psychic self. I don't know just imagine. Angels are the silent selves of people that have suffered but are unharmed. Maybe they never came to life.

> Now I hold on to my keys like my life depended on them. Symbolic of something. Fear of being locked out. Left out of whatever is happening. Nothing was as it appeared. A mask over the moon. Life was an eclipse. I was in the dark.

A hole has developed in my head. Holes in space. Holes in the Ozone layer. All matter is disappearing, A black hole. Alice went down a rabbit hole. Everything is disappearing inside it. Keep forgetting things, shopping, numbers, names. Time of forgetting. Black holes eat matter but where does it go. Into nothingness.

A shot in the arm becomes a hole in the head. Last time it was more of headlong spin down. Hell was other people in the rehab centre. All with their own holes, worried sick about everything.

Here and now the neighbours complain about the cherry blossom. Pink pollen carpets the streets and the delicate fragrance is only detectable in the early morning. I smell the petrol fumes coming through the window. I complain about the cars. Leave the cherry blossom alone my heart cries out.

Feeling sorry for myself. No-one else will. I want to be creative but it just won't come so I can indulge in self-pity for a while. It's depressingly fun. So many stories in my mind waiting in the line.

Sila Tarina

The vital beginnings of writing have been discussed. In Chapter 3 we turn to more how-to-write ideas, and choice of writing materials. A journal can provide a container for diverse types of writing. Thinking of expressive and explorative writing as keeping a journal can make it seem practical and reasonable to try all kinds of different forms, hopping and skipping between them at will. All within the safe yet challenging confines of the journal.

WRITE!

1. Begin every session by writing for *six minutes* with no given subject. Allow the hand to follow the flow of whatever appears on the page: you will find subjects to write about appear on their own: if they don't, then describe something about your surroundings, or that you feel.

2. Write your name at the top of a clean page: first name, middle names, family name. Write whatever comes into your head about any aspect of it: in note form, for five minutes. This might be memories from a long time ago, or things you've read about the meaning of your name. You can't write the wrong thing: put it all down; you might surprise yourself.

3. Draw your lifeline from birth to death. Include all vital life event milestones as artistically, diagrammatically or roughly as you like, on a big piece of paper or several A4 sheets stuck together. It might include *my promotion*, or *when I fell in* love, or *when I met my best friend/wonderful colleague*. Try to write without prior thinking, as far as possible: write whatever arrives on the paper, however divergent or even unimportant it might appear. NOTHING is unimportant in this work. You can cut the paper and stick in new pieces as needed.

4. Look over your lifeline; there will be other things lurking, wanting to be included: insert them, even if means cramming, or cutting and sticking in more paper. You can always redraw a legible version to keep and refer to; and update it over time: vital things will occur to you later.

5. Pick an event from your line. Allow yourself to choose at random, without deliberation. It might be an occasion you know to be important, or you might think: what on earth made me think of that? Don't stop to worry about it: if it's come to your mind, it's right to focus upon it. Write without stopping to think. You might like to consider these questions:

   - When did it happen?

   - Where was it?

   - Who were the important people?

   - What did they say and think? What were they wearing?

   - Which season was it and what was the weather like?

   - How did you and the other important people respond?

   - Why?

   Write for up to 20 minutes or more. Remember you can't get it wrong, and don't worry about grammar, spelling or form; you can always do this later. If you find you've started in the middle, just put the beginning in as it occurs to you. You'll be amazed how much sense it makes.

6. Reread all you've written, including the *Six Minute Write*. I want to ask you to read with unfocussed attention. By this I mean: uncritical

and open to whatever might come to your mind. You might want to add any details or change something (without bothering about rules of grammar, etc. – you can always do this later). You might notice connections between the longer piece and the *Six Minute Write*: if you do they're useful; no matter if you don't. You might jot notes about what rereading your writing makes you think and feel (though it doesn't matter if you don't wish to explore and record this).

CHAPTER 3

The Journal

An Everyday Ally

A personal journal is the most trustworthy friend or colleague possible: always available for any confidence, moan or query, to offer constructive solutions, and never destructively critical. It can clarify and disclose possibilities, knowledge, skills, experiences, previously forgotten memories. This chapter introduces many writing strategies, and makes suggestions about user-friendly notebooks or folders.

Much more goes on in the human mind than is ever normally used; much of it crucial. *Key* writing pays full attention to thoughts, ideas and inspirations, some of which might be surprising. One new writer commented: 'it unlocked a secret I didn't know I was keeping from myself'. This writing goes down on the page as if bypassing the normal thinking processes, almost halfway to dreaming. Just as we run speculatively through a dream on waking, we can read and reread this writing for what it has to tell us from the other side of the usually locked door.

Anne Frank called her journal 'Kitty'. Locked in a tiny space to keep her safe from the Nazis, Anne had no other best friend. She poured her heart out to her dear diary, never imagining that by a series of lucky chances the world would be able to read it long after her brutal, untimely death. Anne's journal is full of girlish ideas, hopes and fears, as well as heartrending facts; Kitty was a secret confidential companion at a time of need.

Writers really do keep notebooks and journals. They really do sit on hills, beaches, in cafés and bed scribbling thoughts, ideas and inspirations, often leading to novels, poems, plays. This exploration is open to everyone, however, not just published writers. Here is a poet's journal extract shortly after her mastectomy and her mother's death:

I'm weeping today – for myself because I'm afraid of dying. I get up for dinner. I could lie in bed drowning in tears for ever and that won't do. My night was so bad it extended into the day. Manic images of the hospital.

Oddly I feel released from my mother at last – this is my body, different from hers though the disease is the same, my scar embroidered by Mr Jones. And my own fight which I can do – not under her shadow.

Alicia Stubbersfield

THE THINGS: WHAT TO WRITE WITH AND ON

Writing materials are significant. Different equipment is likely to create different writings with very different impacts.

My notebooks are ordinary book size, with pictures on the cover, usually bought in art gallery sales. I choose slim ones as I don't like my hand perched above a bulk of pages, and anyway I love starting a fresh new one. For many years I always wrote on bigger loose-leaf paper. I liked being able to slip pages in and out at will, inserting letters, news-cuttings or other things which took my attention. I also liked not having a special volume with me always. What made me change? I only know that I now love the neat containedness of my notebooks. I carry a smaller one with me everywhere, and transfer useful thoughts or observations into the bigger one later. Constantly needing new notebooks provides family and friends with straightforward present-giving possibilities, too.

My choice is to write with a soft pencil with a rubber on the end. A pencil whispers over the page, and can be rubbed out immediately (though I generally scribble out hastily if I don't like something). A sharpener is always at hand to give a maximum chance of clarity, since even I sometimes can't reread my own writing. I love rubber-ended pencils so much they are the only things I am a kleptomaniac about. The pencil I am writing this with now was provided for a meeting at an organisation in London; it is black sprinkled with silver oak leaves and acorns, with a rubber on the end: I confess to taking more than my allotted one of these beauties before I left.

Ahmed was locked into a bullying work relationship with a colleague with whom he worked day after day. He'd heard how writing can be helpful and stayed on after work to try it out at his computer on his desk. Yet he found it depressed him more and more, as he always wrote the same destructive moan. He came to me for help as he had decided he had no other option than to resign his senior position. I felt it was the lack of open exploration and constructive writing strategies which stuck him in a destructive writing spiral, and suggested various strategies, one to do the *Six Minute Write*, followed by one of the methods listed below.

Another vital change was to leave work early and go somewhere he'd never been before and write there. Ahmed worked in the City of London, and took the tube (underground train) out to its furthest reach, Epping Forest. With him he took a cheap spiral-bound reporter's notebook and a fistful of coloured pens from the conference room at work. He sat under a tree listening to the wind in the early summer leaves overhead and wrote stuff he would never have written anywhere else. What he wrote enabled him to perceive that although he couldn't change the bully, he could change his response. He used writing to work out how to alter his way of being with the bully, who was eventually confounded because the victim was no longer a victim but stood up for himself.

Different people choose different materials. Some prefer the keyboard; this doesn't work for me, as seeing my words on the screen in measured print makes me itch to turn it into ordered text with proper grammar. Furthermore I feel distanced from my words; creating them with a pencil, they flow from my body. I have seen people use bright pink fluffy notebooks, tiny kiddy pads with cartoon covers, big business-like dark-coloured A4 perfect-bound books, suede-covered artists' sketchbooks, school exercise books; and loose leaf folders of all sorts, from leather zipped folders or ringbinders, to flimsy patterned cardboard. Paper is all sizes, and white blank, white lined (close-set lined, or feint broad ruled), continental squared, or coloured. I used to go to sessions with a pile of coloured paper, fan it out and invite people to choose a sheet and coloured pen: and write indigo (cerulean, cherry, vermilion, primrose, etc.) thoughts. One doctor keeps a pad of yellow paper always in her car shelf and desk drawer, close at hand for when the last patient leaves. She writes her way back to understanding, clarity and peace of mind.

A cheap notebook and coloured pens enabled Ahmed to begin writing. Such materials can give a sense of lightness to the enterprise, or childlikeness even; what's the need to get it right and proper if the materials are cheap? Pencil, since it can be rubbed out, can give a sense of creative redraftability.

Computers can be good because anything can so quickly be deleted; yet they can give too much of a sense of final proper text on the screen, especially if it underlines inaccuracies with red or green squiggly lines; *Key* writing seeks inspirational leaps, not grammar and final sense. A computer furthermore, being a machine, can be felt to mediate unhelpfully between writer and writing. Writing flowing physically from the body through the hand can be facilitative. Many well-known writers still handwrite notes and first drafts. It's just as well, as they donate their manuscripts to museums for posterity: computer drafts are overwritten and lost.

As a child I was given little hardback books by my aunt for Christmas, with days of the week marked out and a tiny gold clasp and key. No-one, not even my aunt, showed me how to write in them, despite having eminent diarists in her ancestry. So after the first few days of the new year, my beautiful diary remained closed and clasped. A blank notebook, or paper, is for me to put date and time, and scribble for as long or little as I like, and as often or seldom as I like. I found my preference for what I wanted to write in changed over time. One journal keeper orders piles of identical notebooks, a sort he's used for years, and keeps full ones in neat rows on his bookshelf; another writer writes on anything which comes to hand and doesn't keep it carefully at all.

HOW TO WRITE?

The *Six Minute Write* (Chapter 2) is always a valuable opener, even when I think I know exactly what I want to write about. This is writing whatever comes to mind without question; not stopping to think; not consciously using any writing rules.

Sometimes this scribbling can seem to be nonsense, even a waste of time. I was taught that all writing should be purposive; it should be carefully planned and focussed. So over the years I've tussled with a scolding schoolteacher or parent who seemed to peer over my shoulder ready to wield their red pen. My experience of many years of writing with such permissive flow, for six or more minutes, has taught me how it'll suddenly veer towards startling insight. Nobody else need ever read this scribble, it is mine; if I redraft the insightful passages into material I want to share with others, there's no need for them to know about the rubbish dump I dug from.

My desire is to write my style, any style, anything, anytime, anywhere, anyone, anyhow, anyway about everything or nothingness. What an amazing journey. Writing a diary is completely different from writing for medical journals – it is for my personal pleasure without the intention of leaving a mark in the professional literature. I can write it my way, using my own style. No one will tell me whether I am right or wrong, good or bad, appropriate or bad taste. It is just 'me' and I can be me and express myself. It won't get rejected. I won't get hurt. This kind of writing is perfect. I am my own editor. No one tells me what to write except my hand. When I write, my heart is impatient while my mind is wondering what my heart is up to. My hands scribble spontaneously and my eyes just follow.

Yvonne Yi Wood Mak

Here are a set of approaches I've found useful, both for myself and others:

Lists

Lists are a good way of doodling, allowing words to take a walk onto the page on their own. Requiring no punctuation or grammar, they can resemble, or even become, poetry. Lists can be of absolutely anything, such as: Things I really like (or loathe); Things I do not like touching; Things I collect (e.g. objects, recipes, friends); Objects I own but would rather not (think widely). More challenging lists might be: Lies I've told or acted out; Ways I've been insincere. A list of such as What I loved as a child (e.g. sweets, puddings, toys, things we did or people said) might lighten a gloomy moment.

Kathleen Russell, an Episcopalian priest and lecturer in ministry in the USA, used writing to help her with a daunting project:

I felt a fair amount of trepidation about starting the key work on my doctor of ministry degree; the self-doubt came from my old history of not finishing things because I could not pull off the final writing. So I set myself to make a list of 100 words to describe 'my doctoral project'.

The list started with 'arduous, challenging, complicated', went onto 'a gift to me, a gift to others, an adventure, exploration, the other side', and finally 'blessing, gift, ME, MINE, my handwork – a basket, a quilt, a clutter of abundance, cornucopia'.

As I reread my list, it became clear it wasn't so much about the project itself, but about what it meant to me, my relationship with it. Three images came up: a tinker trying to sell a wagon of wares; Merlin who conjures a new world and gives others (students) entry into something new and fulfilling; and the Mad Hatter (or was I the white rabbit?).

So many of the words on the list were not of fear of failure, confusion, or being out of control. Most were inviting, hopeful and meaningful. I was able to embrace being tinker and Merlin – even the Mad Hatter, who is a little dangerous; he just shows up – like a lot of good learning – it's in the surprises. Through this process of writing and reflection, my relationship with my project changed from one of anxiety and self-doubt to one of trust, ownership and hope.

Kathleen Russell

This list is about going through heroin detox:

Day
Waking Up
Sheer Terror
Dread
Fear of Post
Weather
Do not know what to do
Radio
Housework
Shopping
TV
Silence

Sila Tarina

Keywords

Keywords are ones which have attached themselves for some reason, popping up in the mind sometimes quite out of context. Write the word at the top of the page and write whatever comes in *Six Minute Write* fashion. I've often woken up with one in the morning (the number 4 once, another time 'black': both gave lots to write about and understand). It might be something someone said (dwindle, stockpot, patina were significant for me at different times). Creating keywords can be good too: ask someone else for a word, any word, or open a book, paper or magazine at random and take the first word (an old strategy: people used the Bible for divination in this way).

> All he wants is prestige; he's not interested in research to increase the sum of human knowledge, in caring for his patients, in developing the careers of his team. I looked up the word *prestige* in the Oxford English Dictionary. It means 'illusion, conjuring trick, deception, imposture'. Hmm this really gives me a fresh perspective on this big important professor. I'm not going to be a rabbit coming out of HIS hat!
>
> *Fergal*

Music

Write from the title or some keywords from a song going round and round in the head. Focussing on the tune can sometimes bring some words to mind if it isn't a song: these are the keywords. Or writing with the wordless music playing inside the head can allow words to appear. Music can be an evocation; different pieces of music will start different sorts of writing. Some might be memories: Benjamin Britten's music takes me back to my East Anglian past. I can hear not only the sea but the birds and the wind in the reeds and rushes. The music of my youth, The Beatles and Paul Simon take me to remembered places and events. Here is a man approaching his retirement:

> That tune time and again – what is it?! *The Last Waltz.* Why that? What are the words: 'the last walz will last forever' – pretty romantic. I think it's my retirement! Things seem to be so moving into place for doing all sorts of retirement yet worky interesting things. And I WON'T be owned and directed by any institution: I can say NO, and I won't be tangled up in their politics and personalities. I'll pick and choose and do interesting projects and just keep on working in the way **I** want to, with the people I want to IN MY OWN TIME – 'the last walz will last forever'.

Hmm – might not be that though – might be me and Leah: once we're retired we won't be pushed and pulled around by institutions and work – we can waltz forever – until the end of time.

Samuel

Doodles and diagrams

Doodles and diagrams (e.g. flow charts, networks, graphs) are also openers and extenders. Visual representation of thoughts can be invented appropriate to the time and task. *Spider diagrams* (also called mind-mapping, clustering, brainstorming…): write a keyword in the centre of the page and allow ideas, concepts, images, any words at all to splatter over the page, all connecting to the central word like a web. On rereading, they will seem to cluster illuminatively. Different coloured pens can influence what happens too.

Observation

Observation through all five of the senses can develop understanding. Noticing detail enhances pleasure in surroundings because it extends awareness. It also enables closer perception of the nature of people's expressions, interactions, and therefore feelings. It therefore makes us more perceptive colleagues and family members. Tuning in to our world and our people makes us closer to it and them.

In my journal I note something I've observed every day, using all five senses (sight, smell, touch, taste, hearing) and the intuitive sixth sense (intuition, sensing something). Here's an example of a well-remembered smell: 'that house always smelt of home pickled onions: a huge open jar always at the ready in the kitchen'. I wrote the below following a request to write about a container; my container was the lovely ancient Quaker manor house in Oxfordshire where I was staying; I put my weekend observations into the poem. The floorboards I walked barefoot on are in the medieval solar and undercroft.

Charney Manor
The quiet ferments
with the perfume of piebald broad-bean flowers;
the satin of floorboards, warm under naked feet;

the tang of peppermint; and the new moon
low in a silent dawn,
sharp as a well-honed paring knife.

These things weave a spell around women and men
treading a dance as antique as the manor;
but there's no touching – fingertip
to fingertip – in this quadrille,
and the music is the screaming of swifts,
the wind in the poplars,
and the inaudible murmurings of the house.

And then they all leave, the last lingering;
does her bag hold precious manuscripts,
priceless canvasses?

No.
Just an awareness that for five minutes
the only vital thing in the world
can be a thrush in the dappled shade of a sycamore
beating a snail to death
on the lichen-scribble of a grave.

Gillie Bolton

A noblewoman of the tenth-century Japanese court, Sei Shonagan, wrote keenly observed, often cutting comments on her world. Her *Pillow Book* includes many lists, using intriguing categories with which to observe. Under 'Things that are near though distant: Paradise; The course of a boat; Relations between a man and a woman.' She maintains that 'A preacher ought to be good looking. For…we must keep our eyes on him while he speaks; should we look away, we may forget to listen' (p.53). Her many observations include:

one has carefully scented a robe and then forgotten about it for several days. When finally one comes to wear it, the aroma is even more delicious than on freshly scented clothes. When crossing a river in bright moonlight, I love to see the water scatter in showers of crystal under the oxen's feet.

Sei Shonagan (1967, pp.181, 200)

Such minute but inspired observations must have deepened her awareness and pleasure in ordinary everyday occurrences, despite her intensely frustrating life.

Developing awareness of everyday actions can enhance clarity of perception and delight in living in the present. Anxiety about the future can be lessened, and the weight of unalterable past events lifted. It too often takes personal disaster or illness to lead people to realise the value of everyday goodies. People with terminal disease wrote these: 'I never before knew birds sang in winter'; 'I had never before noticed the beautiful shape of a leafless winter tree', 'I had not realised how enchanting it is when little children jump and sing for no reason other than the joy of being alive'. Awareness of the wonderfulness of our fragile life led one to write, 'I don't worry any more. There's only one thing worth worrying about: the illness or death of my loved ones, and it hasn't happened.'

We shouldn't wait for terminal disease to sharpen our awareness and bring a sense of peace. It can be practised by close observation and journal note-taking. Having written about my garden this morning, I felt happy about sweeping up the fallen and blown blossom covering my yard. I'll remember its ephemeral beauty much more vividly when I leave on Monday.

> My wild cherry tree is now pale green, with clusters of brown where the vermilion cherries will grow. The tiny blossom petals cover the garden like snow; yesterday they were blown horizontally by a gusty west wind. Fallen forsythia blossom delineates the edge of the periwinkle bed: bright yellow fringing the dark leaf green, an odd late deep blue blossom accenting the yellow and green. Forsythia blossom also fill the holes in the outside door mat, creating a black and yellow geometric pattern. They have blown in swirls across the yard, bright spring-coloured against the grey asphalt. The young oak still has last year's brown leaves, rustling dryly in the wind. Two blackbirds were tumbling in it yesterday: mating. To the west a neighbour's wild cherry is still clouded with white. To the east, towering near in front of the distant tor, another neighbour's ornamental cherry is opulently pink.

When in London I write about the architectural surprises I notice from the top of buses, or as I tootle by on my bike. Of more immediate practical use are observations about people and relationships. Invited to a prestigious formal dinner at one of our oldest most distinguished academic places, my host was not as I remembered her, but rather offhand. I examined my conscience in reflective writing: what had I done? Musing in my journal I realised she was a shy person probably under stress at that dinner, with many important people present. I realised it possibly had little to do with me, and was therefore able to be relaxed and as much myself as possible at our next meeting. Relieved to meet once more the person I had known, I was even more relieved my faithful journal had helped me not to be defensive and apologetic.

Trance Writing

In Trance Writing, Ruth Folit uses a very ingenious method:

> I enjoy using 'Trance Writing', with my eyes closed, in a relaxed, even trance-like state. It's quite relaxing and seems to keep judgment and inner critics patiently waiting in the hall. I'm less demanding of myself, less critical, and more comfortable with letting things flow with my eyes closed. (Because I'm not watching?) It is the essence of what journaling is all about.
>
> First, I do some slow, deep, relaxed breathing to settle in, slow down my thinking brain, make sure my fingers are on the keyboard 'home' row. My head is tipped back, chin jutting up, and my neck and throat are relaxed. At this point I'm quietly shifting to an internal focus, more in touch with my inner space than with my surroundings, and my fingers do the writing, not my brain. I start typing, knowing that there will be plenty of spelling and grammatical errors. I write about half a page or more in this state.
>
> I've also done Trance Writing in bed, with a small keyboard while almost lying down. I just re-read a journal entry which sounds like it was written by a barely literate drunk: misplaced modifiers, a soup of typos, crazy shifts in tenses and viewpoints. However I'm able to re-string my words into a more coherent whole, which not only communicates better with an audience (if I'm writing for one) but also helps clarify my thinking as well. Here's an example, raw:
>
>> Perhaps the morning pages hsouldb ecome eveing pages – squeezing out the worries of the day before going to bed a tnight. Is it a kind

of moving mediation that brings toether my hands, barn and harte into a full-sized unisficaiton, that is ulimted pouring of myself

And, here unscrambled, as a blog post for www.lifejournal.com:

My journal is where I wring out the worries of the day. When I write it's a moving meditation that unifies my hands, my brain, and my heart. It is an outpouring of myself onto the page. The lines and squiggles of ink/pixels are a piece of my truth sitting in front of me. I can read it, touch it, examine it and leave it – and then return years later. Writing brings me peace, brings some rational thinking to my worries, brings together loose ends, and brings to the surface some of the unspoken thoughts and fears that rattle around in my mind.

My journal writing captures the snapshots of my days, which when placed together in sequence, create a flip book of my life. It creates a narrative, a story, and ultimately helps me make meaning in my life. Writing helps me outline the shapes, the edges, the shadows and the light which help define who I am.

Ruth Folit (see www.IAJW.org)

Blogging

A blog is a journal written directly onto the world wide web, shared potentially with an unlimited unknown audience. The name comes from Web Log: rather odd, as a log is a very particular kind of journal including only precise specific factual information like the exact position of a ship at sea, totally unlike the personal, often confessional nature of many blogs. Despite the name, blogs offer the personal writer a responsive community, so they feel less alone and more appreciated and heard.

Journal writing with this public audience is a twenty-first-century written communal conversation. Emails and texts are the other new forms, but blogging openly communicates with both friends and strangers. Writers are often anonymous with fictional names, and readers can write replies in a similar way. Those who write anonymously often give friends, relatives and colleagues their web-address (url) so they can be identified.

I am a Christian with incurable cancer and, to be honest, divine intervention is the only thing that is going to save me. Firstly, the blog is a way of communicating quickly and efficiently with the many church networks praying for me. Funnily enough, having a wide audience is really important to me. I find the thought of people not understanding what I'm going through very lonely. There is something reassuring in knowing that people are watching us, sharing concern and staying in touch. However, if I do die in the near future, the blog will act as a record for my children of what it was like for me to go through the experience.

Mark Halliday

Bloggers, and those who respond, write with and for a community which might include anyone in the world. They gain the satisfaction and support of knowing their vital thoughts and feelings have been registered, heard, and hopefully understood. A teenage girl born with the HIV virus blogged her feelings about discrimination at school, and school-mates apologised after reading it. Mothers of young children, often a lonely time, blog their experiences and receive many appreciative replies from people willing to enter into fruitful discussions.

The mother of a still-born baby became depressed and felt very alone in her bereavement until she discovered the website of the Stillbirth and Neonatal Death Charity. Her friends had been unable to help with her grief, but through the SANDS website she shared her experiences with people in similar situations. She said these are people who know how to grieve, and know how share each other's grief: it's a bleak forum but gives comfort and companionship.

Clarifying opinion or plans

Key journal writing can be sharply focussed upon practical issues when necessary. It can help with decisions which need to be made daily, organising and running events, tackling sticky situations, creating invitations, ensuring a team or family are in the right places at the right time with the correct equipment.

- The checklist servants, or *tin-opener questions*, have served me well for years. Checking through what?, why?, how?, when?, where?, who?, using them as sentence stems, can ensure all essentials are covered.

> I keep six honest serving men
> (They taught me all I knew);
> Their names are What and Why and When
> And How and Where and Who.
>
> *Rudyard Kipling (1902, p.83)*

- Lists can help make decisions such as between job offers or where to go on holiday, or which strategy to use. The simplest is a list for *for* and a list for *against*; adding a third list for *maybe* can be enlightening as our lives and thoughts have huge areas of grey, rather than all being black and white. It can help to give a weighting to each item, such as a number between 1 and 10 (10 being strong and 1 being weak). Often the result is surprising. Even more odd is that often I take a decision the opposite of what the outcome indicates.

- Metaphors can enable hitherto unnoticed feelings and assumptions to surface (see Chapter 7).

- Diagrams such as *spiders* can be useful: several can be written with a different keyword in the centre of each.

- The *Six Minute Write* can help discover lurking theories and inspirations. Often when asked for an opinion, there seems to be nothing to say, or too much too disorganised. *Six Minute Write* type open-flow writing can enable confused thoughts and ideas to be expressed and then rewritten and sorted into a logical comprehensible sequence.

Caroline shows us how she used her journal to help her over a hump.

I applied for a job, had an interview and then had to wait two and a half days to hear. I decided to write down how I was feeling, and didn't stop until I had exhausted all of my thoughts:

Pain. Shame. Fed up. Anxious. Very anxious. Why didn't I say this? Why did I mention that? Should have been more concise, more structured. Feel I let so many people down. Feel betrayed. I was encouraged to apply for it. Now what? Now what do I do? ... Why have I allowed myself to get into this position? Feel a bit sick. And very sad. I could have brought so much to that organisation. Ok, it was a bigger job than I really wanted, and the organisation is on ropey financial ground, with lots to unpick and change. But I would have liked to have had the chance…

The paper was a safe space for me to write exactly what I was feeling. By capturing them on the page I was able to contain them, and the need to go over and over them diminished. Afterwards, if I was tempted to revisit the thoughts, I only had to remember that I had written them down and the need stopped. This enabled me to realise that I could put the situation to rest and move on.

Caroline Hadley

Journal writing can be a way of communicating the most intensely personal things. Many prefer to keep writings completely private, in a form only to be reread by themselves and no other. Many share with writing group, partner, therapist or friends. Some share anonymously with an unknown readership through blogs.

A journal can be a container for any kind of writing at all; there are no barriers. In Chapter 4 we'll turn to more specific vital elements: place, people and things.

WRITE!

1. Begin every session by writing for *six minutes* with no given subject. Allow the hand to follow the flow of whatever appears on the page: you will find subjects to write about appear on their own: if they don't, then describe something about your surroundings, or that you feel.

2. Write a phrase, a line, or as much as you like in response to each of these beginnings. They will help you to observe your present, past and future with all five senses + the intuitive sixth sense. If one seems to want a lot of writing, focus upon that, and return to the others another time.

   • Today I smelt…

   • Yesterday I saw…

   • Last week I touched…

- When I was a teenager I heard…

- When I was little I tasted…

- Tomorrow I will sense…

3. a. Use the framework of 'Today I smelt…', but write your own version: what you heard yesterday at work perhaps, or what you tasted as a teenager (that first kiss?).

   b. Take one of the lines from either of these poems and write more about the occasion, including as many details as possible.

4. Make a list of significant clothes in your life, whether worn by you or by another. It might be school uniform, an interview suit, a doll's dress, a friend's necklace you coveted, something worn for a wedding or other ceremony, a theatrical costume, shoes worn by an admired person you didn't dare approach. Or perhaps a garment you remember and don't know why. If it's come to your mind, it's worth writing about. Write as much about associated events as you can remember, including colours, smells, scenery, what the clothes felt like, what you said or what someone else said to you at the time and so on.

5. When you begin to feel you've written enough, stop and take breath. Then reread the *Six Minute Write*, and whatever of the other writing you've done on this occasion. Read it slowly, gently and uncritically. If there's anything you want to change or add: do. Don't even begin to think about grammar, or spelling, or obeying other rules. You might want then to jot down notes about what it makes you think and feel (though it doesn't matter if you don't want to now).

6. You'll probably stop writing for today. On starting again another day, write for *six minutes* before anything else. You might like to reread today's writing, and see if another event comes to mind to write about.

CHAPTER 4

Place, People, Things

Place affects us enormously, as do the things we live and work with. Friends, colleagues and relatives, as well as foes, can have tremendous impact on our lives. Familiar or remembered objects and places can help us feel more grounded, more secure and confident. Talismans such as a stone found on a holiday beach, a respected colleague's gift of a pen, an always-worn inherited ring, link us to important and stable people and times. This chapter suggests a wealth of ways of exploring these crucial associations.

Writing can strengthen and develop those links, helping to understand their significance. It can open up memories of places we hold dear, locating us even more confidently with the past. Writing in this way gives me a sense of continuity with the me who was a little child, muddled teenager, burdened joyful young parent, anxious new book writer. Unlocking associations of objects, people and place can help clarify my sense of my life's coherence and support a sense of direction, both in my work and home.

OBJECTS

The word souvenir means 'to come into the mind', from Latin (OED). A host of memories and images can be invited into the mind, by a simple object, if written about in a flowing way akin to the *Six Minute Write*.

> This collar-stud was his, of course, bone and brass. I see him standing, leaning back, just home from work on Fridays, growing flushed as his thick fingers wrestle with its intricacies, sighing with relief as he hands to you the strip of sweaty cloth which will be washed and ironed before Monday. Collar-studs, cufflinks, corsets – puzzling concepts that epitomised the mystery of adulthood.

> Thimble, dulled and dinted, but still intact. When you wore it to force the needle through resistant cloth or especially leather I always feared it

would slip and you'd be hurt. But also, I knew it would protect you. I think this ambivalence came from its name. Thimble seemed a flimsy word. But its weight reassured me when I wore it. It didn't suck at my skin like foxgloves, it simply rested there, rendered me invulnerable.

John Latham

What better-known object is there in fiction than *Winnie the Pooh*? This wise 'bear of little brain' and his friends, known the world over, were based on the real stuffed toys played with by the author's son Christopher Robin. Memory-laden things do not need to be still possessed to be written about and their significance understood better, as I found with this writing fragment:

Cuddly was the bear I loved
cuddled so much his fur was bald
the suit I knitted covered him
from eartips to leaking toes
all that showed were beady eyes
and black re-embroidered nose.

He had to go in the bin
you said 'it's either him or me'.

This helped me overcome an odd grief about a teddy bear, which I realised was not odd at all since he was my only loving companion at boarding school aged nine.

Photographs carry vital images and memories. They are the only things which, along with film and tape recordings, offer real tiny glimpses of the past. A photo captures a fragmentary instant of time, place, person and things. Smell-free, silent, tasteless, feeling only plastic, and even colourless if it is an early photo, they also only include whatever the camera focussed upon; rarely the photographer. Musing reflectively in writing on photos – recent or from a long time ago – can yield fascinating material.

Important images might be from calendars or picture postcards of known places. I can be transported to times when I escaped from my hated school by looking at postcards of the surrounding East Anglian coast. I write about marshes and reed-beds, beach-huts, water-tower, lighthouse, and harbour, smell of seaweed and honey-coconut gorse, beach-pebbles crunching underfoot, gulls screaming overhead, taste of fresh fish and chips, and the sea-wind which nearly blew us off our feet. Hella's writing gave her a way into a place of psychological peace at a time of stress following the death of a beloved aunt.

I was sent a card of a beautiful door. It really intrigued me, though I didn't know why. So I asked it to tell me about itself.

Dear Hella, I called you and you came and saw me. You are standing in a long dark dingy corridor, having passed dull doors on the way. And now you stand in front of me. What you hadn't noticed in the picture, is that the door has your name upon it. Open the door, go in and see what you find there.

You put your hand on the doorknob, and fearfully push the door open and look inside. There are lots of things from your life, all arranged for you to look at. You pick up your pen which saw you through all your exams. You're so glad to have it back, and take it with you as you look around at so many other things full of memories. And then you see another door, at the back of the room; unmarked this time. You are braver at pushing this one open; you have to push hard, but are so glad you do.

Inside is the most beautiful room you could ever have imagined: wide, spacious, with a view of the sea rolling up to a sandy beach with soft susurration. You walk in, and think 'here I am, at home'.

You look around carefully and memorise 3 words about the room: peace, calm, width of vision. And now you have to leave. Quietly and gently you step back into the other room, replace your trusty pen, say goodbye for the time being to the other aspects of your life, and return to the corridor. It's no longer dark and dismal; two of the doors you passed previously now look quite inviting; you resolve to return and open them.

Take the memory of that lovely room, and those three words which bring it vividly to mind. Life is treating you so harshly now; you can find solace, rest and hope there, in your mind: 'peace, softness, width of vision'.

The Door

Dear Door in the picture, I can't believe how much writing about a simple card has given me; thank you. Through all the painful bereavement I am going through, I have been able to bring that room back to my mind at any time and find peace softness and width of vision.

Hella

FOUND OBJECTS

Other things can valuably set writing off as well as objects and places with direct personal significance. Road signs can give unintended messages. I regularly cross a railway line, main road and river on one of my walks. The railway stile has a bold sign: *Stop Look Listen*. I reflect upon how vital this instruction is, not just for writing but for life itself, and have put these three words at the top of a page, and written below in the *Six Minute Write* way.

Altered Priorities Ahead is a road sign I've used as another writing cue. I look out for words in public places, on packages and bottles, seeking messages. All except the title of this was found on cleaning materials' labels:

Sex
Creates shine and sparkle
CAUTION
Keep out of the reach of children
Rinse hands thoroughly afterwards
Avoid prolonged contact
May release dangerous gases
Recap tightly after use
Can be irritating to the eyes
If symptoms persist consult a doctor
Extremely flammable

Gillie Bolton

I found a key in the street once. Writing in my journal I worried how its owner got into their home or office: that led to a story about being locked out. Then I experimented with image: it came to stand for the key to my life. I put it on a kitchen shelf so whenever I came upon it I smiled, reminded that things weren't all bleak or difficult. I had the key to unlock my problems: writing in my journal, where I often asked 'what's the solution to this?' There always is one, even if it's: 'come on Gillie, take a more positive attitude!' Eventually I felt someone else's need for my key was greater than mine, and I gave it to her.

PLACE AND PEOPLE

Home on the one hand, and mountains, caves, or icy deserts on the other, are extreme places. Think of Emily Brontë's yearning evocation of her beloved Yorkshire moor in *Wuthering Heights*. Her sister Charlotte described the moor I've spoken of here, her *Jane Eyre* being set in my Hope Valley village. A.A. Milne created a secure bounded environment, the Hundred Acre Wood, in his *Winnie the Pooh* books. I have intermittently written about a tiny room in my student days, attempting to understand the association of the place with the significance of the life experience I had there:

> My college gyp-room, thirty-six years ago. Funny name – just looked it up – gyp means the lowest servant. The gyp-room was a pretty unromantic place – tiny with twin-tub washing machine, sink, iron, double ring cooking-hob. These days there'd be a microwave, I suppose. Ironing my green and blue tartan lawn shirt. Daffodil time of year, dull day: there were no windows anyway, only a skylight. Like a flash of sunlight I knew how much I was in love, that I would only ever feel that way about one man. Innocently ironing my own shirt, and my life suddenly and unexpectedly changed forever. What does it mean – that happening in the room of the lowest sort of servant – very funny!

Writing about people from any period of life can help in understanding their importance. If their impact was negative, understanding them better can help heal nagging guilt, hate or fear associated with their memory. I suggest thinking of someone important from any period, who hasn't been seen for some time (they might even be dead), perhaps family, friend, older adviser, colleague. Describe these:

1. Where they were; in what setting or place.

2. An object associated with them.

3. Something they often used to say.

4. A mannerism or way of being.

5. Something about them a bit mysterious or unknown to you.

6. A vital question you would now like to ask them: what is it?

7. Write their reply to this question.

Sue Sims' father, and her relationship with him as a child, is described through a very lovingly created scene. As a way of writing about a significant person, it is both very touching and effective.

Brass Rubbing
A roll of black paper,
from the attic,
unfurled
and held in place with books
reveals a knight in armour
complete with sword
and in some other place
just out of sight
of fairy tales
a man and his girl child
kneel in awkward intimacy
in a cool stone crypt
rubbing at brass

creating a joint masterpiece
that has yet
to be laden
with the weight of memory

Sue Sims

Jonathan writes about what it's like working with so many people in his profession. He's chosen a deceptively simple-seeming form which disguises a very serious message about his work: this comes through clearly at the end.

These are the stories doctors tell:
The Christmas gift, the troubled gaze,
The cognitive decline of age,
The family rift, the loss of sight,
The ones who lived, and those who might,

The dying and the worried well;
These are the stories doctors tell.

And these are the patients doctors know:
The tired and anxious, the slow, the lame,
The ones that never go away,
The bright, the angry malcontent,
The addict and the one that's sent,
The garrulous, and those brought low;
These are the patients doctors know.

And these are the moments doctors fear:
The unexplained, the shadowed lung,
The relative who asks: 'How long?'
The purple rash, traumatic birth,
The contemplation of our worth:
Examinations that draw near.
These are the moments doctors fear.

And these are the journeys doctors make:
The drone of dusty lecture halls,
The teaching round, the nights on-call;
Uncertainties and things un-said,
The visit to the hospice bed.
That one mistake. That touch of grace.
These are the journeys doctors make.

Jonathan Knight (2012, p.26)

It's hard not to write about people; we're pack animals who make lasting bonds and allegiances. However vital our homes, offices, possessions, it's people who ultimately matter. Whether the examples in this chapter were written in response to a place or thing, they primarily concern people. Chapter 5 looks at a fundamentally human way of communicating: by stories.

WRITE!

1. Begin every session by writing for *six minutes* with no given subject. Allow the hand to follow the flow of whatever appears on the page:

you will find subjects to write about appear on their own: if they don't, then describe something about your surroundings, or that you feel.

2. Draw a lifeline.

   a. Take a large sheet of paper or stick several end-to-end. You could continue on the one you made for Chapter 1 *Write!*, if there's space.

   Put in PEOPLE who have been important to you in your life. If you add them into the original lifeline, you could use a different colour. They might be such as my work partner, Uncle Tom, Glyn Jones the music teacher, my boss, as well as the novelist Jane Austen, or singer Paul Simon.

   b. Pick a significant person from your lifeline. Write a letter to them, telling them about your life now, and how important they were or are to you.

   c. Write their reply.

3. Insert vital PLACES in your life and work (or make a new lifeline). Once more – allow your hand to pick its own – try to include as many as possible. Use a different colour again if you like.

4. Now important OBJECTS in your life. Be creative!

5. Pick a place, object or person from your lifeline.

   a. Write whatever comes about it, her or him as openly and freely (i.e. like the *Six Minute Write*) as possible. Write as descriptively and fully, putting in details, as seems right, perhaps telling a story.

   b. Choose another to write about afterwards perhaps.

6. Choose an object important to you. Hold it, put it in front of you, or see how clearly you can remember it, if you no longer have it. Describe it fully. Write about associations and memories it has for you.

7. Write an account – reflective or story – with the heading: *The Gift*.

8. Reread all your writing to yourself: the *Six Minute Write* as well as the others. Read and alter in any way you wish, openly and uncritically.

CHAPTER 5

Tell Me a Story

Ask a colleague about a stormy meeting, they'll tell its story; ask anyone about their illness or bereavement, or a birth, or ask a child about a picture they've drawn: it'll be told as a story. Narrating our stories in writing is even more powerful.

WHY STORIES?

People are as full of stories as champagne bottles: the cork might be difficult to ease out at first, but, once started, there's no stopping the fountain of delicious fizz. We tell stories all the time to help make sense of experience. Writing them can enable deep reflection upon our lives, their meaning to us and the sense they seem to make. Writing the stories of our lives can help create coherence, and support us in understanding better.

We tell stories about our lives and the lives around us: over cups of tea, meeting carafes, pints of beer, glasses of wine. We also eavesdrop through films, television, the news, magazines, literature: the fascination is partly in seeing how others tussle with, and respond to, life. We narrate experiences and events, and our thoughts and feelings concerning them on email, letters, notes.

Greater sense can be made out of life dramas if I can pick out a narrative line to write into a story with a specific plot (my first chemotherapy; another meeting with that dreadful director; Tommy's first tooth…). Who said what, and how I felt about it, and what it led to me saying and doing can be aired and thought about. Other elements fade into the background, such as what other people were doing, saying and thinking at the same time and place, as well as what I was thinking about other issues. These come to the foreground as a different story later, or a retelling of the same story from a different perspective.

Before starting as a General Medical Practitioner (GP) I had finished off my training with a six-month job in genito-urinary medicine. For a convent-educated girl this had been rather challenging but by the end of the job I was proud of the matter of fact way I could deal with all manner of embarrassing conditions. When, therefore, in the first weeks of being a GP a slightly nervous man began the consultation with 'I think I've got warts Doctor, my wife had them first…', I eased into my previous role without difficulty. 'Right, fine' I said briskly 'Just pop behind this curtain and slip your trousers down'. At first I took his hesitation for shyness so I flashed him my most reassuring smile and gestured to the couch. He walked across slowly, sat on the edge and said 'But they're on my hands, Doctor'. Suffice to say he never came back to see me.

Writing this story has helped to reframe the experience from a completely excruciating one into one which if not exactly my proudest moment at least demonstrates an ability to see the funny side of misfortune. Pomposity is one of the ever-present pitfalls of working as a doctor and sharing stories such as these is a powerful antidote to it.

Helen Starkey (2004, p.93)

Recording and reflecting upon significant life events can be vital for older people, particularly if the stories are written. This can help knit together the continuity of their sense of themselves. I am the same person as the little girl who loved riding my grandfather's cob, Kitty, although she was so fat and I so little that my legs stuck out at right-angles. The word *record* comes from re-, meaning again, and -cord, meaning heart. I live or tell my heart again each time I record one of these stories onto paper.

WHAT IS A STORY?

Stories have satisfying shapes, generally with beginning, middle and end, and tend to concern particular identifiable facets of people, situations and places. Life as we live it, conversely, is all middle; and all rather a muddle with different stages of different plots cutting across each other, and inconsistent people and situations. Apart from individual births and deaths, life events go on and on and on, in and out of each other in an unsatisfactory unfinished way. An individual death might be the end for one person, but come at the beginning or middle of surrounding plots, involving different people.

Stories, however, with their satisfying form, involve people, an initial situation, and a development of that situation, leading to a slightly (or very) different state than at the beginning. That's the basic; most stories also involve a particular place and a specific movement through time. Writing suggestions in Chapters 2 and 4 involve drawing lifelines and inserting vital events, people and places. Characters, events, place and time are the building blocks of story.

Writing a story intuitively, in an unfocussed *Six Minute Write*, rarely, however, involves thinking through the involvement of characters, plot events, location and chronology. Because we story-make intuitively, the pen can be put on the page, or fingers on the keys, and these elements will naturally appear in a coherent narrative form. Some stories are concise; some go on and on, entrancing or boring listeners or readers. I emailed one yesterday:

> My sister and I saw a wedding as we passed Southwark Cathedral on Saturday. The very black groom wore a black suit and the blonde bride a frothy white frock and veil. The black women guests all had HUGE wonderful hats; the white ones wore tiny plumes of feathers or big bows in their hair. We then went and bought cheese and bananas at the market under the railway arches.

Out of quite a cast of characters, only two are central: my sister and myself, and a subplot of wedding people. The place is distinctive: Southwark Cathedral and Borough Market on Thamesbank; as is the time, a busy Saturday. The chronology is finite: about half an hour. The plot development: the two major characters were much amused and intrigued by the spectacle they chanced upon; they undertook some satisfying shopping. All the other plots, subplots, characters and situations of that morning were eliminated from this tiny story.

It gives the reader a sense of: a convivial sisterly outing; the multiracial character of South East London; the busy nature of this bit of the Thames south bank where the cathedral is on top of the market (or the other way round I suppose); a colourful picture of a traditional British custom. It tells my reader something about me: I like to take time to stop and stare through railings at things going on. Writing such as this at the end of an email means I receive similar snippets of other people's lives in return; sometimes from people I'll never meet, such as copy-editors.

WHY STORIES?

We tell and write stories to communicate: to tell others about our lives and to make it clear we'd like human contact in return. People are social animals and constantly affirm and reaffirm their role and place with each other, and seek positive feedback about actions, experiences, thoughts, ideas, values, principles. All around me here in central London I hear a constant chattering buzz: people walking, sitting, standing outside bars, in person, on mobiles. If they're not talking they're texting. And behind the many office, college and home windows more people are meeting, emailing, faxing, telephoning, lecturing, teaching...

People also tell stories to listen to themselves: reaffirming themselves to themselves. Locking my bike outside the supermarket yesterday, four older ladies were discussing their surgical operations. It was clear they were not listening to each other, but each rehearsing their own account. They probably do this time and again. People need to grasp the narrative of their lives: 'I am the person who has had a new hip and is just venturing out of the flat for the second time in three months, and it feels exciting and a bit scary'.

Another day it might be: 'I'm the person who's just become a granny!' or 'I've just been kissed by a cool guy!' or 'the child I diagnosed as having a head-cold nearly died of meningitis; the parents are furious: what am I going to say to them?', 'I went to sleep in a meeting and snored loudly', 'I've just been made redundant/had my house flooded/been diagnosed with cancer/lost my mother'. All these major life events cause reassessment of future life projects and possibly values; they necessitate a rewriting of personal life narratives. Talking about them on the street corner, in order to rehearse them to oneself, is not going to be enough; talking about them with a trusted colleague in the pub is probably insufficient for the more major life events. Writing about them, reflecting upon that writing, and possibly discussing those reflections with a confidential other, and then perhaps rewriting or writing some more, might be enough. In my work with doctors, I found that early experiences were extremely significant and have far-reaching effects on later practice; here is Seth's:

The Unequal Struggle

She sat day after day on her mattress, clothed in a tattered and dirty dress, giving me a shy smile as I did my rounds. She had been brought in from God knows what village or hovel. The hospital was full and she was accommodated on a mattress on the floor in the corridor. She couldn't walk because she was paralysed below the waist. There weren't any relatives or visitors. She was about 14 years old.

After a while it occurred to me that I could get her a fresh dress from the 'calamidades', the bales of clothes that came apparently from Scandinavia to our part of Mozambique. I saw people with Stockholm University on their chests. I saw Michael Jackson. I saw a gaunt, bony woman hoeing the dry dusty ground in an 'Iron Maiden' T shirt.

So I acquired a clean, fresh, bright print cotton frock of roughly the right size and took it to her in her corridor. When I held it up in front of her and she realised it was for her, she leaned forward and embraced the skirt of the frock, somewhere in front of my knees and laid her cheek on the material as if she were caressing a lover.

I wrote this as a recollection some ten years after it happened. When we in the comfortable world hear the seemingly endless bad news from Africa, I am reminded of this incident. It exemplifies for me the type of human misfortune that lies behind statements like 'Mozambique belongs to that group of countries known as Highly Indebted Poor Countries'. Those are people's lives we are talking about, the only lives they have.

Seth Jenkinson (2003, pp.51–52)

Why *write* stories if we tell them daily? However much we talk with others, it's sometimes not enough. Some issues need much reflection and discussion; the biggest need massive amounts of airing. Because writing gives the story a physical presence on the page, rather than disappearing on the air with the breath, it can give more satisfaction. It can of course still always be rewritten in a different way, fixed differently on a further piece of paper another day, and even again and again.

Writing a story can draw out elements we don't know we know; one beginner wrote, 'things come out because the story lets them out'. Writing is initially private, unlike conversation: the page silently accepts anything. People write about their own lives, bent over the page trying to scribble as fast as the words appear, not fully aware of what they've written until they reread. This isn't only in the nature of writing rather than talking: it is also the creative process. Sculptors, painters, musicians as well as novelists and poets say how they do not direct what their hands are doing; the art *seems to make itself*. 'Where did that come from?' people often ask bemusedly when they read their writing back to themselves.

A reminiscence of times past might be wanted for grandchildren to read in the future. A story written is a story remembered on the paper. It can also have greater impact on both writer and reader than a spoken story, perhaps because it's a created thing in their hands to be read, reread and referred to.

Writing can help people tell different perhaps more challenging stories than the well-known, fairly safe ones they tell orally every day. Some people always put themselves in the best possible light: things go wrong only by chance, or are someone else's fault, and so on. Some are the opposite, and tell stories in which they are forever the victim, or put themselves down in some other damaging way. Creating genuinely enquiring personal stories can be unsettling: careful boundaries are needed when they're shared. Writing can offer a safe enough space for personally challenging stories to be experimentally created.

DEVELOPING STORIES

Writing about work and life events can challenge the status quo, or highlight atmospheres, unacknowledged disagreements, discomforts, hesitancies, queries. HOW a story is told can be rewritten. My Saturday morning wedding story was intended to be light, sunny and observational. I could, however, have told about: race, local politics (Borough Market might be bulldozed and developed), history (site of Shakespeare's original theatre), family tension. I do write some of these: in my journal.

Everyone has often-repeated work or family stories. I've often either written the story as I remember it, or written about it being told by its habitual teller (my mother or my boss). I then give the story a title. In my family we had stories I could call The Wrong Key, The Chinese Bad Luck Mask, and Grandfather's Will; in my work, The Bullying Belittling Boss. These stories became unquestioningly stuck in the way they were always told. Yet I've found that each and every story can be rewritten from the point of view of a different colleague or family member, one who does not figure much in the original story perhaps. It's a strange adventure getting inside the story, encouraging it to retell itself in a different and insightful way. I don't generally tell the person I'm writing fictionally about; though sometimes it has led to useful conversations we really needed to have.

POINT OF VIEW

Point of view, fundamental to story, can be played with in writing. Altering the perspective can challenge what the story is about. My sister would have written my Southwark Cathedral wedding story differently from me; so would the bride, the groom, or the Italian cheese market-man. Here is a family doctor (GP) needing to listen to her patients better:

> I was so angry with her. Can't she see the little girl needs to be in hospital, getting the best care and treatment? I was shaking when she left, just wanting to shout at her in her smug confidence; she's so wrong! It twists my heart so to see a little one in a wheel chair; if that was my child I know what I would do.
>
> Then I knew I had to do something about my rage, and remembered something a trainer had said about writing. So, when yesterday evening everyone happened to be out, I sat in the garden with pen and paper feeling rather a fool. But I started to grasp a different perspective after the first line; the change was extraordinary.
>
> I wrote as if I was the mum: 'It's love she needs now, the love of her parents and brother in our own home. Nothing can save her; she has so little time to live, we want to make it a time to remember forever.'
>
> How could I have been so arrogant to think I knew better? I realised I didn't know that I would do differently if she were my child; perhaps if I loved someone like that I would do just the same. I'll approach these cases so differently now. And if I ever feel so certain of my own view again, I know I can rely on writing to help me out.
>
> *Shamini*

A story is a sliver of life, whether fictional or based on a personally experienced event. A snapshot excludes the photographer and other people and things beyond the perimeter of the photo, smells, sounds, tastes and touch; a story excludes similarly; a story writer can ask questions such as: from whose point of view have I written this?; how different might it have been from the point of view of another?; what didn't I include and why?, what might the other people in the story have been thinking or feeling at the time? Or, in sharing the writing with a trusted other, they might ask such questions and be able to discuss it constructively.

This story was written by the daughter of German Jewish refugees from the Second World War. Superficially about knitting, it's also about belonging, culture, confidence, taking charge of one's own life, and many more issues.

Knitting our Stories

I struggled with English knitting, I dropped English stitches, sometimes smuggling the knitting home in my school bag so my mum could make it better, but I was found out.

On the teacher's desk was a pair of giant knitting needles and a large square piece of knitting in lime green string. Plain knit, no purls, no stocking stitch. Every time one of us dropped a stitch we had to stand out there in front of the class and knit a row of lime green.

I often stood there, six years old, scabby knees and grubby socks one up one down. I worked the needles painfully slowly as I attempted to reach the end of the row with all my stitches intact. At the end of the term the teacher presented me with the green object 'a dish cloth' she said, '*you've done most of it, take it home to show your Mother*'.

My mother was the creator of pink wool dresses, soft jumpers with scalloped edges and fluffy striped scarves, the knitter with flashing needles. They knitted the continental way, the women in my family, holding the needles close together whizzing up and down rows. They chattered away: foreign sounds and foreign laughter. Continental afternoons, with continental cakes, continental knitting, only the grey English drizzling winter outside the window.

I walked miserably out of the school gates, I tried to tear the lime green apart with my teeth, but the yarn was stringy and hard, I slipped into a nearby driveway and hid behind a tree. There was a patch of earth in the shade; I dug into this stranger's flowerbed with my bare hands, like a little puppy burying a treasure, me burying the shameful object, the secret of my failure.

With much struggle, and the help of the internet, I am now, having just turned sixty, a proud continental knitter, my yarn confidently on the left side, as the women in my family knitted before me. I have earned my rightful place on the *knit and bitch* sofas of the new multicultural age of English knitters.

Carry Gorney

As Carry shows us, stories are knitted into our lives. Writing them, as well as knitting them, is important. Poetry, which we turn to next, is our other natural form for communication, especially at times of great need.

WRITE!

1. Begin every session by writing for *six minutes* with no given subject. Allow the hand to follow the flow of whatever appears on the page: you will find subjects to write about appear on their own: if they don't, then describe something about your surroundings, or that you feel.

2. Write as openly and unthinkingly (as close as possible to a *Six Minute Write*) as you can to any one or more of these titles. Include as many details as occur to you; you might write six lines, six or sixty pages:

   - A time I learned something from experience

   - An event which was unexpectedly successful

   - A puzzling episode

   - The secret

   - My secret place

   - The other side of the wall

   - Off the map

   - A chapter from my memoires

3. Think of a significant journey in your life, anything, from 'my first holiday to Cornwall' through 'my first lecture abroad', to 'my adventure in the Siberian wilderness'. Tell the story but focus particularly on one particular incident in as full detail as you can. Include dialogue between the characters, description of the place and description of one character, and so on, as you wish.

4. List some significant times of change in your life, such as going to big school, first day of the new job, meeting a particular person, the birth of a child. Choose one to write about in as much detail as you can.

5. You have won a prestigious award, and have been asked for a brief description of your life and achievements, to be published in a national newspaper. Write this in about 200 words. Give it a title!

6. Reread all your writing with unfocussed attention. Alter or adapt as much as you wish, responding uncritically and positively to the writing.

CHAPTER 6

Poetry

Poetry writing can express what we need to say but cannot yet bring ourselves to say aloud for others to hear. Poetry's conciseness enables it to reach the parts that prose cannot, leaping straight to the heart of the matter. Poetry is an exploration of our deepest and most intimate experiences, thoughts, feelings, ideas and insights: distilled, pared to succinctness, and made music to the ear by lyricism. For some, it is the only way to explore and express certain things, directly diving for the heart of the issue, with no messing around with sentences and grammatical rules: a way of saying exactly what I want to say, and finding out what I need to say. Jeanette Winterson found insight and solace in poetry as a child, saying, 'it isn't a hiding place, it's a finding place... The poem finds the word that finds the feeling' (Winterson 2011, p.40, p.187).

This chapter shows how poetry can give form and shape to vital thoughts and feelings. Written, these things are still silent yet not dissipated on the air like spoken words. The bigger experiences are in life, such as trauma, the more difficult they are to speak, the more they need to be expressed, and the more other people find listening difficult. The ancient Greek philosopher Aristotle described the powerful effect of poetry on people's emotions.

The first draft of poetry writing can enable thoughts, feelings, memories to tumble out of the body via the hand, onto the page. The poet William Wordsworth said, 'poetry is the spontaneous overflow of powerful feelings'. One of my reflective writing professionals said, 'I like poetry because I can't make it do what I want. It has to do what *it* wants.' Redrafting can enable further understanding. Another student was amazed to find she got clearer and clearer about what she thought as she redrafted her poem.

> Journalism is what people talk about in public
> Novels are what people talk about in private
> Poetry is what people think and feel, but don't say.

Poems 'profoundly alter the man or woman who wrote them', observed Welsh physician-poet, Dannie Abse (1998, p.262). Every poem teaches its writer something they didn't know they knew. It's odd how we can know so much and not know we know. Poetry writing can drag a fishing net through the mind, trawling for what is there. It can show an original way of looking at or understanding something. It can help make sense of and accept a feeling or experience. It can be personally illuminating.

Creativity itself can be transforming. Making something as satisfying and expressive as a poem can make me feel differently about myself, loved ones (and others), significant events and my surroundings. A poem is a work of art on the page: the white spaces around it like a silent frame. Poems have been likened to pictures in words. Making something always makes us feel better. It can also help take our minds off worries or anxieties.

'Poetry has the capacity…to remind us of something we are forbidden to see', said the USA poet Adrienne Rich (2006). This illuminative power comes partly from the way ordinary things we've taken for granted become different and even strange. It can also make unknown distant things seem ordinary and graspable. Wordsworth made an expanse of daffodils magical, showed us how their memory enabled reflection and joy later in life. Poetry can help us feel more in tune, more connected with our world.

Instead of feeling fear and disgust for the down-and-out on the street, John used close observation and empathy to help him understand better and feel compassion:

Man on Street Corner with Blanket over Head
But doctor, I see better in the dark…
Dark is where my mother's face
re-forms out of her ashes,
grows young, bends over me.
Doctor, let me be. Dark
is where I look
into my lover's heart: and see.

John Latham (2006, p.21)

Poetry is halfway to music, always a rhythmical soother or stirrer of spirits. Poetry, like speech, does not necessarily come in sentences and paragraphs; and they share an ability to leap from one subject or image to another while still making sense. Poetry is the form of choice for many at a time of personal need (bereavement, loss, retirement, anger, falling in love) because it is so satisfying to throw emotions rhythmically onto the page without having to complete sentences, and without having to fill each line from beginning to end. The page can capture the emotion, holding it safely outside the mind.

We use poetry to say something we want or need to say, but can find no other way of saying. Poetry must have said *I love you!* for millennia, as well as *love is overwhelming, scary, destabilising, creates jealousy.* Here are two of the oldest known poems in the world.

Love shook my heart
Like the wind on the mountain
Rushing over the oak tree.

Sappho (Balmer 1996, p.55)

In love beware:
a scorpion waits
under every stone.

Praxilla (Balmer 1996, p.26)

Big emotions can make us speechless. Feelings, such as love whether of a lover or a child, despair perhaps during war, horror like at 9/11, grief as at the death of a parent, are difficult to express. Adrienne Rich said, 'every poem breaks a silence that had to be overcome' (2006). The words, charged with a force of needing to be said, seem to appear from nowhere onto the page; unexpressed, they can build up and harm.

Soldiers wrote poetry in the First World War. Ordinary lads, had they not lived through such horror as the trenches, they would probably never have written anything other than the odd letter and list, certainly not poetry. Yet that succinct expression of feeling and experience, allied to the comfort of words arranged musically, gave them a priceless outlet. It also enabled them to tell us of unspeakable events years later. Listen to this simple cry of pain at losing a good comrade.

Lost in France: Jo's Requiem
He had the ploughman's strength
in the grasp of his hand.
He could see a crow
three miles away,

and the trout beneath the stone.
He could hear the green oats growing,
and the south-west wind make rain.
He could hear the wheel upon the hill
when it left the level road.
He could make a gate, and dig a pit,
And plough as straight as stone can fall.
And he is dead.

Ernest Rhys (2002, p.179)

Poetry can communicate ordinary things, making them seem wonderful, startling even. Descriptions of nature can make both writer and reader aware of something they'd always seen (heard, felt, smelt, tasted), but never noticed. Putting myself in contact with my surroundings by writing poetry always makes me happier because it takes me out of myself, helps me forget whatever anxieties, fears or miseries might otherwise be in my thoughts. All these years later I can sense Rhys' distress at the loss of his friend, and the balm of creating this limpid picture of Jo, an extraordinary ordinary person, and the countryside he lived and worked in.

BRINGING POETRY INTO DAILY LIFE

Becoming absorbed in creating poetry can chase away negative thoughts; poetry writing can fill the mind so that it crowds out anxieties, fears and even pain for the time. Its two constituent elements both have this power. One element is the initial thought-free *Six Minute Write* which can tell us about what we think, feel and remember, and help us to understand our relationships to other people and our world. The other side of poetry writing is the intense focus upon redrafting the few words gleaned from the initial *six minutes* into the best possible order and shape. Here is a lawyer on the struggle between work and home:

How can a mother an attorney be?
With a little child always pressing at her knee
Begging for a story and a comforting cuddle
The mom's mind seeming always in a muddle

The mom comes home in disarray
Having had a very busy day

Her nerves are frayed
From being in the courts
There are bills to be paid
And she's out of sorts
Life seems abridged –
Only an hour 'til bed!

Melanie Fein

Poetry can say a lot in a few words. Here's a method I use. I look back at some *Six Minute Writes* or any other personal scribble, and take a brief bit that seems to be important. It sometimes has meaningful images in it; poetry uses image, particularly metaphor, to a great extent. I then copy it out in short lines, leaving out some negligible words like 'and' and 'the'. I then read it aloud and alter words or word order to make it sound more musical but still make perfect sense. As far as possible I use my ordinary language and normal mode of speech; language was used differently when poets such as Tennyson and Coleridge wrote, and I can't copy their style. This fiddling about with the words and their order seems to help the poem communicate what is there inside me needing to be communicated – with myself. After doing this for a long time, it's then ready to share with the right person in the right way at an appropriate time, though I do keep some totally private, and never share them with anyone.

Sometimes I take my personal journal, pencil and pencil sharpener to a particular place: the local park, my kitchen, a café, by a river, and note whatever I can see, hear, feel, smell, taste. Then I reread it and choose bits I like best and make them into a list of phrases, all shorter than the page width. Having fiddled around with these lines, shortening them and choosing words which best describe what I perceived, and which sound more musical, I type it up, reread it and work on it a bit more as poetry always looks different once copied out. The poem *Charney Manor* was written like that (see Chapter 3). Here is a healing poem, written after Tom's mother's death.

My father, Robert
Waiting silhouette, white and with hunched back
White stick, white coat and white beard,
All colour drained.
I am finally proud to take his arm

Touching his arm at the end
Brought together by the pain
Of watching his life's love slip away
We come away from the cold crisp hospital bed

Tapping and clasping each other in the corridor
The nurse could not meet our eyes
I didn't tell him it was the sister from the ward
But he knew by her clipped footsteps

When my children leave
Will I have the skill to let them go
And wait for them patiently to come back
And take me by the arm?

Tom Heller

Another method is to think of a person important to me, listing elements about them which come first to mind. *Jo's Requiem* by Rhys is a list. The poet Elizabeth Barrett Browning started a list poem with 'How do I love thee? Let me count the ways' (1993, p.62). My poem might be observations (Gran always smelled of baking; Gran was as round as a hug), or things I felt (I felt safe in Gran's kitchen). As with the observation poetry, I read the list and cross out the least important, then re-order it so it feels more satisfying. The person begins to appear before me, and I always see them in a new light, understanding them the way they think and feel (or thought and felt), and their importance to me. Here's the beginning of a poem, John describing his newly dead son:

An almost grin – self mocking
as if you'd been caught out
playing some silly trick…

John Latham (2006, p.75)

Poems can be about anything we want or need to know more about. 'The early evening midsummer moon was like torn tissue hanging above the moor.' Writing that gave me a sense of nature's tremendous power because I know the moon's a vast lump of rock poised over the earth. I had been feeling sorry for myself, yet this contact and closeness with something unknowable, ageless, took me out of myself, comforted. Another writer, trying to come to terms with boarding school memories, suddenly understood what cooked onions made him think of. His poem was about secreting them under a loose floorboard all one term. The thought of that rotting smelliness hidden under there made it impossible for him ever to eat onions. Poems can enlighten us about anything.

RHYTHM

The sound of words matters. As human animals we live our lives to a natural rhythm: the heartbeat of poetry and its sister music bring us comfortingly close to that. Poetry draws on other life-rhythms such as the daily round from sunrise to sunset; the pull and draw of the sea deeply affects us when we are near it. Normally rhythm is subtle, though some writers prefer to build the poem around the way it rolls and rattles along, or surges like the 'shining big-sea-water' in Longfellow's *Hiawatha*. My children's favourite bed-time poem, this is an exciting adventure with a happy homecoming ending to most chapters, and a soothing dancing heartbeat running throughout.

> By the shores of Gitche Gumee,
> By the shining Big-Sea-Water,
> Stood the wigwam of Nokomis,
> Daughter of the Moon, Nokomis.
> Dark behind it rose the forest,
> Bright before it beat the water,
> Beat the clear and sunny water,
> There the wrinkled, old Nokomis
> Nursed the little Hiawatha…
>
> *Henry W. Longfellow (1960[1854], p.27)*

Here, Alicia uses more ordinary speech rhythms to write about her mother's death:

> I've beaten cushions, thrown books at walls,
> broken milk bottles in complete despair
> before becoming expert at silence.
>
> I want to see my anger like a meteor
> gloriously exploding into particles,
> disappearing at the slow light of dawn.
>
> *Alicia Stubbersfield (2006, p.34)*

Originally poetry was recited because most people couldn't read or write. Spoken to music, or made to sound as musical as possible, it was a pleasure to hear and remember. Repeated sounds also make memorable rhythm. Homer's Odyssey, written well over two thousand years ago, has repeated phrases like: 'rosy-fingered dawn crept up the sky', or 'they rowed over the wine-dark sea' (1996). Listen to Tennyson (1993), writing a gloomy scene using repetition of 'eee' and 'ooo', 'mmm', and 'nnn'. At the end, when the Lady dies, there are five final-sounding 't's at the end of lines ('Camelot', 'boat', 'afloat', 'wrote', 'Shalott'). It sends a shiver down the spine. When he wrote it Tennyson must have needed to explore and understand melancholy, fear and suicidal angst.

> She left the web, she left the loom,
> She made three paces through the room,
> She saw the water-lily bloom,
> She saw the helmet and the plume
> She looked down to Camelot.
> Out flew the web and floated wide;
> The mirror cracked from side to side;
> 'The curse is come upon me!' cried
> The Lady of Shalott
>
> In the stormy east-wind straining,
> The pale yellow woods were waning,
> The broad stream in his banks complaining,
> Heavily the low sky raining
> O'er tower'd Camelot;
> Down she came and found a boat
> Beneath a willow left afloat,
> And round about the prow she wrote
> *The Lady of Shalott.*
>
> *Alfred Lord Tennyson (1983[1842], p.82)*

CRAFTING POETRY TO HELP UNDERSTANDING

There must be as many ways of writing poetry as there are people who write. Some only write at a time of extreme emotion, like bereavement or confusion in love. Some write more often, using the form to express feelings, thoughts and memories, without re-writing. Many others wish to search for the set of words which come as close as possible to whatever they're trying to evoke from their mind, heart and spirit. It's a search for how to describe the look in her eyes, the exact quality of grief on turning up the old photo, or what the fear was like when for so many hours after the bombs I didn't know where he was. Bringing memories and images into clearer focus, by redrafting, can support healing insight.

Redrafting is exacting, yet absorbing: delving and experimenting, listening to the words. This grappling with language, and with memory and observation, this playing with words, is compulsive and exciting, just as any hunt. We were not born to have everything provided in a supermarket. People were stone-age hunters and gatherers for millennia, and have only been civilised for a few thousand years. The thrill of the hunt, or the search for elusive delicious roots, fruit and berries, has been replaced by many things in our culture, but few more satisfying and less damaging to others as poetry writing. It's a way of feeling really alive, and a first-class antidote to anxiety and depression.

A notion exists that poetry, in order to be 'real', must spring out of the writer as complete and finished as Eve from Adam's rib. Poetry is what we want it to be. If a personal and vital telling of experience is wanted, perhaps only for the self or a few others, then natural undrafted poems are perfect, and often of immense value. Redrafting is exacting and time-consuming, but the resulting poem seems as fresh and clear *as if* it had just flowed unchecked from the pen. W.B. Yeats said poetry is only worthwhile if it appears as if the result of 'a moment's thought', however much 'stitching and unstitching' we've done (1903, p.18).

Editing is a final stage akin, I think, to the pleasure some gain from crossword puzzle solving, or Scrabble, absorbing and diverting of attention from anxieties. The satisfaction of creating something as perfect as we possibly can is great; the process can also be soothing because it is so practical (a bit like gardening or cooking, if you like them). The poem is complete as far as saying what I want it to say, and seems to be rhythmical enough. But it needs grooming to be as gleaming and polished as possible, and to communicate as satisfyingly well as possible (the placing of a comma can completely alter meaning). Listen to this fragment; imagine how different it would be without that extraordinary image of 'wrinkled sea' 'crawling', and the second comma:

The Eagle
He clasps the crag with crooked hands;
Close to the sun in lonely lands,
Ring'd with the azure world, he stands.
The wrinkled sea beneath him crawls;
He watches from his mountain walls,
And like a thunderbolt he falls.

Alfred Lord Tennyson (2007[1851])

Editing a poem is similar to grooming a horse. This involves the regular sweep of the brush over warm flanks, teasing out of mane tangles, polishing of hooves; it means most of all quiet communication with alert twitching ears and intelligent eyes, and closeness to the beating of a big trustworthy heart. This is the stage when the poem becomes mine entirely: it tells itself again in my head, and I know it needs a comma here, the deletion of *but* there. It becomes mine at the same time as it takes wing and becomes a thing in its own right: a fully fledged poem which communicates with any reader out there. This ownership, and being able to let go, of one's own creativity is life-enhancing.

This range of poetry writing experience is essential. No-one would want, or could cope with, the adrenaline-rush of the hunt every time they wrote, or indeed the dynamic psychological pummelling of the first stage.

First draft *six minutes* of poetry *writing*, the breathless blind scramble of words onto the page can't really be done to order, whereas one can reasonably readily plan a redrafting, and certainly an editing session. Although the vital first stage cannot be scheduled, it can, however, be facilitated by the regular practice of journal and other personal writing. We learn our own rhythms, needs and wants, and discover ways of setting up appropriate times and places and equipment which are likely to help. We also learn the confidence to know when to give up when writing does not seem to give you anything on a particular occasion: it'll happen another time.

Advice on giving birth
The beginning is the hardest part
but once started
the thing unfolds itself.
Throw in a metaphor or two
to slap it into life

and sometimes if you're feeling flush
nourish it with rhymes,
or, you could let rip
and write a sonnet
but this needs skilled midwifery.
Your labour ends
with birth, a new creation.
And then you have to live
With what you've written.

Vicky Darling

RHYME

So much about poems, and nothing yet about rhyme. Rhyme and rhythm can be really satisfying when they come naturally. Poems do not have to rhyme at the end of lines; too strong a focus on rhyme too early in the writing stages can result in doggerel. Doggerel is verse driven by rhyme and metre rather than the vitality of its significance and meaning. Commercial birthday and special occasion cards offer excellent examples of doggerel:

Roses are red and violets are blue,
Sugar is sweet, and so are you.

Speech is filled with repeated jingle-jangle, hopscotch, hugger-mugger, tit-for-tat arrangements of words. Sometimes they're homely, childishly comforting; sometimes they enforce meaning. Here, in *The Rime of the Ancient Mariner*, the ship is stuck in ice; Coleridge wants to convey intense loneliness and fear of being surrounded by the cold trapping stuff, and the eery noise as it grinds together. He uses vowel repetition (ow, ow, ow, ee, ee). Consonants are repeated: the keening of 'nnn'; the clipped 't's in the first line give a cut-off sense of being surrounded by cliffs of ice. Coleridge was working out a desolate misery, making me feel very glad of my cosy room.

And through the drifts the snowy clifts
Did send a dismal sheen
Nor shapes of men nor beast we ken –
The ice was all between
The ice was here, the ice was there,

The ice as all around:
It cracked and growled, and roared and howled,
Like noises in a swound!

Samuel T. Coleridge (1970[1834], p.12)

Edith found writing strongly rhythmical rhyming poetry a compulsive way of coping with strong emotion: 'I think in poetic rhythm / I dream in poetic rhyme'. Listen to her using rhyme with a satisfying strong explosive sound at the end of many lines:

He was a bourgeois dilettante
A flattering unctuous sycophant
An intellectual neophyte
With the face of a toady troglodyte

With a gut the size of a jumbo jet
A nose like an over-baked French baguette
Cobwebs of fuzz on his parapet
And a whine like an amateur string quartet
He was like nothing you've ever seen yet!

Dancing and prancing – a marionette
His paunch a ponderous silhouette
Always delivering a sermonette
And totally lacking in etiquette
He wasn't a weasel to ever forget

Rarely did he practice rumination
Thoughtfulness or cerebration
Meditation or cogitation
Pensiveness or contemplation
Forethought or deliberation
Intuition or divination
Anticipation or imagination
Obligation or communication

Bereft of an ethical attitude
To lies he gave much latitude
For truth he had no gratitude
Muttering many a platitude
For thinking he had no aptitude

Of verity he was sadly bereft
At telling lies, decidedly deft
Truth and honor he sorely cleft
Of integrity there was nothing left

Edith Darfield

POETIC FORM

Forms like sonnet, vilanelle and haiku can release greater feeling into fewer words, holding emotions firmly within their bounds.

Sonnets

Robert Hamberger says why *sonnets* help him.

Saying My Name
My mother doesn't know me from Adam.
She's baffled by my face, wonders at my words.
I make no sense; but if I tell her who I am
my name might echo down her corridors
to a room where she sits by open windows,
looking up from empty hands to find me there.
She'll hear Robert because of course she knows
those syllables, familiar as a prayer.
It's worth a shot. I say it like a stone
dropped into her lake to test the water,
to see if bubbles ripple from my tone.
Nothing this time. I name my sons and daughter,
say her sisters' names, tell her all our news
to ease the silence, darkening like a bruise.

Robert Hamberger (2008, p.37)

I've used sonnets to write about being in love, childhood memories, my first kiss, Kurt Cobain, a pig, a car crash, a peace march, my children, losing a tooth and about grief as well, particularly the loss of friends, and my mother developing Alzheimer's. They've been a way of discovering some semblance of order or meaning through my history.

The pre-arranged rhyme-scheme over fourteen lines feels like a 'life-belt': searching for a rhyme or half-rhyme helps me find a path through my feelings. Writing poems, even free verse, is often a bit like solving a puzzle: what does this experience mean to me? How can I express this experience, feeling, or memory, in words? Sonnets set me a verbal challenge that paradoxically might help to set me free to speak. For example, love can feel like happy (or unhappy) chaos; a sonnet creates a sense of artificial order through my contradictions.

Robert Hamberger

Pantoums

Here is Lizzie who had heard that writing in form can help with difficult subjects, and so tried a *pantoum*. Her poem is followed by an extract from her journal.

The Shroud

I have grown taller by walking with trees
In pursuit of myself
I lived as a wild one
Sickness an ardent lover stalked me

In pursuit of myself
In icy waters I swam trailing a shroud of grief
Sickness an ardent lover stalked me
Above the stars chimed immortality

In icy waters I swam trailing a shroud of grief
Numbness and emptiness were my friends
Above the stars chimed immortality
Through the dark woods a fragment of moonlight held my hand

Numbness and emptiness were my friends
I lived as a wild one
Through the dark woods a fragment of moonlight held my hand
I have grown taller by walking with trees

Lizzie Chittleboro

The last two weeks I have been so helped by writing poetry. The inspiration has come in the night like hoardings at the station: each one a bright image that jumps up and down and demanding my attention to be chosen. Sometimes they are like a neon light flashing with bright lights in the dark. I choose the brightest one, the noisiest one which refuses to lie down and through writing I experience a sense of peace and release. Like stars guiding me in the right direction as I travel through a strange country.

At the time I was still writing about my feelings after my loss of career and 'shroud' seemed too strong a word to use. I tussled with it for several days taking the word in and out replacing it with 'cape'. It was only as I began to talk about the poem that I came to understand how appropriate the word 'shroud' was. It gave me access to a much deeper level of thinking about the loss which I was exploring. I found myself talking about the impact of the death of my sister on my life. I had found an important key to my recovery with implications for my well being for the rest of my life.

Lizzie Chittleboro's Journal

Haiku

Haiku is a tiny Japanese poem form which traditionally depicts a life-enhancing experience of nature. They are obsessively absorbing to write, because of the precise form. The first line contains five syllables, the second seven, and the third five again: seventeen syllables in all. An aspect of nature has to be evoked (a butterfly, blossom, frog), and then its impact on the writer described or hinted at in those few syllables. In my haiku here *depression* has a double meaning: a state of mind and a shallow hollow in a rock. It's a hopeful poem: life-giving rain *will* fall, and a clear reflective state of mind *will* follow harrowing depression.

> in a depression
> of rock after heavy rain
> a clear pool settles

Poems are so full of images, particularly metaphor, they wouldn't work without them. Metaphor is a jewelled key to explorative and expressive writing, because it can communicate the difficult-to-express, creating something out of often agonising nothingness. We couldn't begin to explain the joy of new parenthood or the despair of recent bereavement without them: Chapter 7 shows many ways of finding and using them.

WRITE!

1. Begin every session by writing for *six minutes* with no given subject. Allow the hand to follow the flow of whatever appears on the page: you will find subjects to write about appear on their own: if they don't, then describe something about your surroundings, or that you feel.

2. Read through your *Six Minute Write*.

   a. Underline all objects or activities: choose one. Or think of a favourite object or activity. Or choose from this list: boot, rat, playing in snow, Cinderella, having a bath, kissing, the wedding, a doorhandle, colleague's/dad's/mum's/gran's/my kitchen/workroom, heavy rain, a loved one's photo, walking by the river, the baby's shoe.

   b. Focus closely on the thing or activity, forget everything except for this. Most of all forget you are writing a poem. Describe it *without saying what it is*, without using the keywords (e.g. *baby's shoe, walk* or *river*).

3. Use the same object or activity, or choose a fresh one.

   a. Write as if you ARE it: write in the voice of the shoe or riverside walk.

   b. Describe what your function is: why you exist (e.g. 'I make you listen to water running over stones instead of the noise of your worries').

4. Make a list of perhaps 20 items, each beginning with 'How...' (such as 'How does the dog always know when I'm miserable?', 'How can I relax at night and go to sleep happily?').

   a. Reread your list with attention, adding or altering any. Respond to as many as you can, or perhaps develop the questions more, or explore around the issues.

   Your list might be a poem already; or choose some elements and change others to make it more poem-like.

b. Write similar lists, beginning with 'Why…', 'What…', 'Who…', 'Where…', 'When…'

c. Choose one or more to write more about at more length, in an open free-writing way, perhaps.

5. Reread all your writing, and make any alterations you wish. Seek only words which accurately give what's in your mind; if you can replace two words with one better one: do. Cut out any words you feel are either extra or reduce its musicality and rhythm. Copy it out so the lines don't reach the right-hand page margin. Read it to yourself aloud (when you're alone) to give a feel for its sound.

6. Experiment with different titles. Experiment with all the words, remembering you can alter anything you don't like: be bold.

CHAPTER 7

Pictures in the Mind

Metaphors

*Metaphors create links between what
we know and what we feel.*

JUHANI IHANUS

Human minds find it easier to grasp things than abstractions. A doctor will be helped to understand the nature of pain when told 'it was a stiletto knife in my forehead'. And these give insight: 'he was a real mouse at the meeting, humbly content to nibble dropped crumbs'; 'she was a panther, waiting silently, poised for her moment then pouncing with irrefutable argument'.

Metaphors can be golden keys to insight and understanding: 'The great muscle of metaphor drawing strength from resemblance in difference' (Rich 2006). A metaphor is one thing described in terms of another (pain = a knife stabbing), which help us into the sometimes inaccessible world of abstractions and feelings. This chapter shows how we use them illuminatively every day without realising; it also offers methods for consciously exploring and experimenting with them; they are a cornerstone of poetry.

'I haven't the foggiest idea what a metaphor is!' a business student stated confidently. Yet the metaphor of a vague idea as being cloaked in fog is effective. He was looking at the subject even worse than when driving through fog: he didn't even have the confidence of knowing the unseen road is ahead.

These business students were clearly *stumped* by being asked about metaphor. A cricketing term, I don't know exactly what *stumped* means, but as daughter and sister of cricket enthusiasts I do know a stumped batsman is out. Once the students realised the effectiveness of the unwitting *fog* metaphor, they began to be happily un-stumped (though I think cricketers can't be un-stumped): they began to understand what a metaphor is.

Metaphors can clarify any abstraction; science and mathematics use them routinely. A chemist, Kekulé, solved the mystery of the chemical structure of benzene when he dreamt of a snake with its own tail in its mouth. In a very few words, or small visual images, metaphor vividly gives a concrete, comprehensible picture. Jane Wilde, who has a significant leadership role, wrote a poem about watching a heron standing completely still 'on a stone in the river' before it lifted its wings and flew away 'gently with ease'. She said of the poem:

> I'd been away a long way to a different place, and when I returned, the contrast could not have been sharper. I came back to the start of a busy work programme and felt disequilibrium. I wrote this to express my need to reflect.
>
> *Jane Wilde (2003, p.43)*

Likening one thing to another brings both into the mind at once: doubling, and therefore illuminating, the mental images.

A young woman was trying to make up her mind between two job offers. She wrote, 'If the two jobs were animals what would they be? The one in Somerset is a rabbit, an owl; the Wolverhampton one is a snake, a rat.' She took the Somerset job because her writing told her she trusted the people and valued the thoughtful small company family ethos (rabbits have large families, she realised when she worked out why her writing hand had come up with that animal).

We sometimes describe ourselves as if in water: floating, weighted down, or even sunk. She was high; he was low; 'I'm only middling today'; the patient was under anaesthetic. Since nothing has physically moved, these are all metaphors. Colour is used similarly: a black mood; she saw red; green with envy; purple prose; a jaundiced (yellow) view of the world; a white lie; baby blues (depression after a birth); and so on. A deliriously happy man at his second marriage 'experienced moments in all colours' (Annie Proulx 1993, p.355).

Deliberately choosing our metaphors can give authority and even power. I wouldn't like to *hit the ground running* with a new project. What do *I* do? I *take wing*! Flying, I can travel up and down as well as along, and there's no ground to slow my winged feet. Flight means freedom: freedom to be dynamically original as well as effective.

Karol Silovsky, a busy general and emergency medical practitioner, wrote about his complicated and frustrating drive to work; on discussion he realised the journey was a metaphor for the whole of his work. Later he wrote about life being a journey, including this: 'At each crossroad there are choices, and at times you wonder whether the choice you made was the right one. However you are where you are. At the end contentment and acceptance, you can always get off the merry-go-round. Or can you?'

My mother always said 'I'm four sheets in the wind' when she was in a muddle: I think she thought of washing blowing off the line. Mother never sailed, but the image she unwittingly used depicted her as a yacht with four sail ropes (*sheets* in sailing language), flapping wildly out of reach, and the boat about to capsize. A pretty accurate description of my mother much of the time.

Mother used cockney rhyming slang too, from her father and where she worked in the East End of London:

sister: skin and blister
wife: trouble and strife
stairs: apples and pears

When I was little I liked climbing the apples and pears to bed, as apples were my comfort food.

Lucy likened *Key* writing (see Chapter 2) to 'a jack-in-the-box opening up to reveal itself' and 'a water lily opening in the summer sunshine to reveal its inner beauty'. Now listen to Lizzie:

At a difficult time in my life, I found the use of metaphor valuable to enable me to express *my* feelings. This poem was the first of a series in which I was able to explore my feelings around leaving work. I researched the word ibex as I was surprised that I had chosen it and found it was thought by the ancient Greeks to have healing properties. Here is part of my journal, and the poem:

I took myself off to clear my head, as I walked I was able to name my fears. I woke this morning with images tumbling through my mind. As I wrote, the power of metaphor enabled me to release from deep within painful thoughts and exchange them for positive and strengthening images. (Journal)

I am a stagnant pool
I would like to be a bubbling brook fed from a mountain stream

I am a heavy itchy overcoat
I would like to be a gossamer scarf light as air

I am a meal of dry cream crackers eaten without water
I would like to be a fresh salad full of colour, flavour and nutrients

I am a dark damp cellar full of abandoned objects
I would like to be a light airy room with beautiful paintings on its
    walls

I am a gloomy, foggy night
I would like to be a fresh sunlit spring morning

I am a funeral dirge
I would like to be a jazz piece full of mellow tones and ingenuity

I am apple blossom bruised and trampled under foot
I would like to be a jasmine flower sweet smelling and luminous at
    night

I am a dead tree rotting in the soil
I would like to be a tall palm tree its face thrust up towards the sun

I am a rhinoceros nearing extinction wallowing in the mud
I would like to be an Ibex leaping from rock to rock

Lizzie Chittleboro

Later, after Lizzie had written many more poems and a fairy story, as well as
dialogues and unsent letters, she wrote:

I remembered these lines:

I am a damp dark cellar full of abandoned objects. I would like to
be a light airy room hung with beautiful paintings. On waking this
morning I had an image of an empty room swept clean. (Journal)

Metaphors can take us by surprise; meanings creep up on us giving insight
into what we think, feel or know. Mice, panthers, cricket stumps, ropes,
sheets, gifts, wings, apples, colours, and so on, all seem innocent until they
are allied to something we need to know more about. The poet Gerard

Manley Hopkins said: 'kingfishers catch fire, dragonflies draw flame' (1953, p.28). Metaphors make ordinary elements of our lives suddenly catch fire and draw flame. Hopkins continues, 'As tumbled over rim in roundy wells stones ring' (1953, p.28). Metaphors not only enable meaning to catch fire and draw flame, but they ring out this enhanced meaning and significance loud and clear, just as the roundness and depth of a well magnifies the sound of a dropped stone.

CLICHÉ

Old well-worn metaphors become clichés. If a picture in the mind is like penetrating oil, clichés must be like corrosive acid or rusting water: clogging and jamming the lock. Clichés can lead to listeners or readers not attending, switching off (to use another cliché) because the words have lost their power of association and are dead.

Metaphors used unthinkingly have power over how people run their lives, particularly working lives. For example, a new employee is often expected to *hit the ground running* as soon as they start; there is no time for new colleagues to get to know each other's strengths and weaknesses and best ways of working together. The word *hit* is violent, and the idea of *running* from the very beginning is exhausting, unreflective and indicative of merely taking up a given role. Team members complain if their bosses *change the goalposts*; within this sporting metaphor is the assumption that employees expect to work to rules created by others, to aim their goals within *goalposts* positioned by their bosses; this is not a discursive organisation where individuals have a say. Employees are sometimes enjoined to make a step change rather than a gradual change in improvement in effectiveness such as productivity. Since step change refers to the shape of a line on a mathematical graph, with this metaphor people and their work are perceived as elements in a two dimensional diagram, rather than human beings.

We can change the metaphors we use, and in doing so change our attitudes. Our bodies are often referred to as machines: people get *geared up* or *change gear*; *coast in neutral* (I wish they did more); *kick start* themselves (too often); need *their engines tuning*. Doctors are written of as *fixing* the body or mind. Gardening metaphors could be used instead. A *germane* thought, idea or initiative would be dynamic and successful, seeds being powerpacks of energy. Only needing water, seeds grow with tremendous power: dandelion seedlings readily push through tarmac. I'd like to burst out of the seed pod, put out new shoots to the sun, and roots deep into the earth.

A powerful way of taking more authority over life, particularly at work, is to listen for habitual metaphors, reflect on what they indicate, and if possible do something to change them.

INSIGHTFUL METAPHOR

Experimenting in writing with the mental pictures which illuminate daily life can enable deep and significant understanding. Our metaphors and other figures of speech can be chosen in keeping with our principles and values. A hospice physiotherapist wrote:

> my work is like spreading compost over the soil, offering advice, exercise, support, a whole mixture of things and then just like the worms work away with that through the winter pulling it into the soil to enrich it so people can use what they are offered and work away with it incorporating it into their daily life and hopefully bring some good.
>
> *Helen Evans*

Light can be cast on what you think and feel about a relationship. A woman had problems with the noise her neighbour in the flat downstairs made. She felt she couldn't approach such a loud, arrogant, vulgar person. Her writing helped her see it was jealousy which prevented her from communicating. It made her look again at her neighbour and see a confident woman in sexy clothes, careful makeup and styled hair. And it made her take a more critical look at herself. She reached this insight by writing sets of pairs – ordinary everyday things – writing them quickly without thinking. They were such as horse and cart, sock and shoe, needle and thread. She then chose these to work on:

> Ms Flat C and I are:
> A button and buttonhole: she goes right through me
> A horse and cart: she's the horse pulling
> A knife and fork: she cuts, I just feed
> Ham and chips: she's succulent ham, I'm greasy chips
> Cat and mouse…
> I think I'll become a mouse if I continue this, and scuttle into a hole in
>   the wall.

With the help of a good friend she was able to call on 'Ms Flat C' in a confident low-key way, finding her to be a nice person who hadn't realised she was causing offence. Writing pairs like this can give insight into a relationship with one other person, you and a client perhaps, you and a relative, friend or business partner.

Another way to be in touch with your well of understanding and knowledge is to become aware – through writing experimentally – of seemingly irrational likes and dislikes, and other significant actions. We don't remember everything we have done or that has happened to us. There's so much to remember, and our minds try to keep darker memories out of daily consciousness. Yet all our memories are there, and they can make themselves known in strange and often unexpected ways.

A man wrote his way through fear of feathers and hens, and disgust at eating eggs. He traced it back to a childhood trauma: although hens were not the cause, they were present and became the image which stood for the whole trauma. Eggs and feathers were therefore feared, because of what they represented, although they were not and are not themselves intrinsically damaging. A woman wrote at length about having to scrub herself again and again until her flesh was raw. The scrubbing was a metaphorical cleansing of childhood abuse which she could not get out of her mind and body, although her memory had forgotten the events. Learning details about the meanings of these metaphors gave these people greater insight and peace of mind. Whole painful memories were not brought back to consciousness thankfully: just enough awareness to bring understanding.

Thinking of things or actions as metaphors can illuminate present actions as well as memories. We often don't understand all our motives. A married man had a developing relationship with another woman; she then married, breaking off the relationship. He gave her an ornamental doorstop as a wedding present, unaware that, with this gift, he was asking her to keep the door open, despite her marriage. Writing about this was painful for him, but it helped deal with his remorse and guilt as well as grief at losing the relationship.

Poetry and metaphor making are as old as writing itself, and so are letters. Conversations in writing, they are our way of communicating when the spoken word cannot be used, for whatever reason. All sorts of letters can be written and replied to in *Key* writing, as explored in Chapter 8.

WRITE!

1. Begin every session by writing for *six minutes* with no given subject. Allow the hand to follow the flow of whatever appears on the page: you will find subjects to write about appear on their own: if they don't, then describe something about your surroundings, or that you feel. Starting in this open enquiring way can pay dividends.

2. Create a list of metaphors:

   a. Think of someone you know well. Put their name at the top of the page (they need NEVER see this writing, though of course you can share it with them if that seems right).
      Write responding to the list below: if this person were an animal, what would they be? Write phrases or sentences, such as 'a great roaring hungry bright orange and black tiger', rather than merely 'a tiger'.
      If the person you've named were an:

   * animal, what animal would they be?'

   * piece of furniture, what would they be? (armchair, stepladder?)

   * food

   * weather or season

   * colour

   * drink

   * insect or sea creature

   * plant

   * child's toy

   * make up some of your own categories.

   b. Reread your list to yourself, alter it in any way seems appropriate if necessary. Extend some of the items, making them more descriptive, or choose one to focus upon. Write as much or as little as you like.

3. List metaphors or other images you habitually use, or hear in your everyday life and work.

    a. Jot them down wherever you are when you hear them. Be aware of the groupings they tend to belong to (e.g. currently there are a great deal of market/commerce, sporting and mechanical images).

    b. Pick out two images which particularly strike you. Write openly in a *Six Minute Write* way about each, noting down anything that occurs to you.

    c. Study your list again: take another one at random. Create a spider diagram (Chapter 3):

    - Write the word (e.g. goalposts) in the middle of a blank page.

    - Allow different ideas or images to scatter themselves over the page.

    - Choose one cluster of words and phrases to write about further in a *Six Minute Write* way on another page.

4. Develop some stronger alternative images for yourself, in keeping with your values and views, like my likening myself to a seed instead of a car.

5. Reread all your writing. You might remember more things to put in, such as smells, touch or taste.

CHAPTER 8

Letters

Life and work push and pull at us all the time, sometimes violently. Writing can help make these forces apparent, as well as offer strategies for dealing with them. This chapter suggests two letter-writing strategies. The first is exchanges intended never to be sent (some would be impossible to send). These can offer insight because addressing a significant other directly, yet knowing they'll never read it, can be liberating. Also writing their reply can be a dynamic fictional exploration of unnoticed assumptions, as well as a way of expressing emotion.

The second way of using letter writing concerns ones designed to be sent. These can be valuable additions to talk: writing can sometimes communicate things people cannot bring themselves to speak. Drafting and redrafting letters (or emails or other written communication) with a high emotional content can also be very valuable. Anger, for example, can be thrown onto the page safely if you then reread and redraft until you reach a version which you feel happy to send. The emotion can be expressed and dealt with in the drafting.

UNSENT LETTERS

Important, tragic or painful events happen, difficult decisions need to be taken, problematic memories intrude, scary tasks need to be done, and problems faced. Of course events such as bereavement or job loss cannot be altered. But there are times when we assume 'life's like that!', when it needn't be. Certain taken-for-granted forces *seem* to direct life. Working out what they are, where they've come from, what can be done to strengthen the positive ones, and get rid of or at least ameliorate the damaging ones, can give greater personal understanding and authority. Here are a pair of letters from Steve, written in a substance abuse treatment centre:

Dear Santa,

This is the first time I've written a letter to you in many years, and in the interim much has happened to me…

All I ask is that the growth I am starting to feel continues. I know that nobody else, including you, can help me to find out the true me – and grow to love myself. My request is, therefore, that I continue on this path. I know then that I stand a good chance of finding that elusive character that is me. I have a feeling that when I find my true self – and grow to accept and love myself, the rest of the things I could ask for are likely to follow.

I hope and pray that you can help with this plea.

Yours sincerely, Steve

Dear Steve

I cannot guarantee that you will continue on the path you are currently on – for that would be to dictate the future. What I can tell you, however, is that as long as you stay in your strength – and in the current vein, your true self will be revealed to you and you will be more aware and accepting of who you really are…

Finally, self-truth, self-acceptance and self-love are the goals for which you are aiming. You are right in saying that as you grow and learn these things, you will be able to love others in the way you've always thought you should – your wife, your children, your family and friends.

Stay safe my friend and treat yourself with gentleness, dignity and respect.

Yours Christmassy, Santa

Steve

Letters which will never be sent can explore different aspects of a situation, paying attention to each. They allow different elements of oneself to surface, be expressed, and understood better. Novelists or playwrights invent characters out of themselves, with the aid of close observation of others, or research. This technique can be borrowed to discover or invent characters who represent significant elements of oneself, to listen to with attention. Here is an amputated leg being addressed as *you* as if in a letter, as a way of coming to terms with its loss.

Phantom Limb

...
But you haven't gone.
Like a child not wanting
to go to bed, you hang around,
tease me with your tricks,
make me try to put you in a trouser leg,
...and just in case I might forget you
you give me
sharp twinges in the foot,
an ache in the calf,
disconcert my ideas of space.

...

Writing gave me some sense of detachment from my own problems and helped me adopt a positive attitude. I was in a way looking at myself from outside and so was able to come to terms with what had happened more easily than I might. My physiotherapists asked to see my poem and have displayed it in their gym to help others.

Derek Collins

Unsent letters and serious illness

Monica communicated with mental illness (she did NOT want to address it as dear).

Illness

You stripped me of myself, tortured me with sleepless nights, shook me until my limbs trembled with fear and filled my thoughts with images of my own death. You killed the simple feelings of being alive – you emptied me of self, and threw me over edges without end day and night. You allowed me to blame myself for losing self, losing purpose, losing a sense of my own goodness. You took away my identity and gave me another one and it was so terrible I can not speak of it.

You are locked away illness and never forgotten and in the dark of night I meet you with flashbacks and fear. I'll never forget you.

Monica

Monica
Each time I came, I departed. Your mistake was thinking I was here to stay for ever. Though the essence of me has imprinted your being, I did not take your life. Think of me as eclipse – the dark overlaying the light – fear made me worse than I might otherwise have been. You know that I came out of emotional and biological imbalance; do not blame yourself for allowing me to enter your life. And do not shoulder responsibility for the chaos that I brought into all the lives affected by me. I stopped short of true destruction. You survived me and you have learned much. I have served my function. And I'm not coming back.

Illness

Monica

Unsent letters and bereavement

A young man's wife died suddenly and unexpectedly, leaving him with broken hopes, and three teenage children to bring up alone. He was offered some professional counselling, but anxieties, hurts, anger and bewilderment kept going round and round, keeping him awake at night and distracted during the day. He wasn't coping and had to take time off work.

He wrote a letter to his late wife, pouring out all he felt, thought, feared, remembered and struggled with. The letter, lengthy, impassioned and exhausting, clearly wasn't one he'd ever send. Although writing helped him understand and accept more, he didn't feel at peace afterwards, but drained and empty.

He then wrote the reply she might have written, without knowing how she would really have replied. He wrote from his awareness of his wife inside him, which initially wasn't easy. With perseverance and deep inward observation of memories of her, he wrote her reply. With it, and with further letters and replies, it became a dialogue bringing greater peace and understanding. He learned: to forgive her for dying and abandoning him and their children; not to beg her to return; to stop saying endlessly 'if only I'd driven her to work that day it wouldn't have happened', and other 'if onlys…'; to stop imagining she'd walk in any day if he did certain things better; to begin to think about and plan a future without her, without feeling he'd betrayed her memory.

Perhaps most important he found a strategy for continuing to be aware of her advice and support, particularly vital with respect to the teenagers. Whenever he was in any doubt or anxiety about them or other issues, he wrote a letter to her in his journal, and wrote her reply. He was able to pour out all his feelings, thoughts, fears, hopes and dreams. Her letters (written by him) were full of wisdom, love and care, combined with lack of criticism: she was brought clearly to his mind every time.

Esther Helfgott wanted to remember life with her husband before he got sick and died:

> Dear Abe
> Sometimes I write letters to you.
> It's a way for me to get to know us better.
> to remember us in the past –
> the way we were
> and the way I thought we were.
> …
>
> *Esther Helfgott (2012, p.41)*

Unsent letters and anger

Anger, and its sister guilt, are two of the elements of *Pandora's Box* most of us would love to do without. Pandora, a heroine from antiquity, was entrusted with a beautiful magical box, but told never to open it. Of course she did, and out flew the world's ills and horrors: negative emotions, diseases, stinging nettles, tsunami waves, and so on. She desperately, but unsuccessfully, tried to jam them back and force the lid back on. Fortunately Hope also escaped from the box, always to ameliorate evil.

Anger and guilt have the volatile force of the contents of *Pandora's Box*. Once erupted, they cannot straightforwardly be constrained back into a recess of the mind, and the lid safely bolted back. Their effect is all too often destructive. Caught in anger or guilt, it's difficult to hear hope's kind voice. The impulse is to hurl the anger at someone, or to wield the guilt destructively inwards: sometimes permanently damaging self-confidence and self-respect.

Anger or guilt – about work, family, friendship, politics or religion – can be spewed relatively safely onto the page, and the letter never sent. We all have a murderer within us: private letter writing can let it out safely. The letter can be reread later and reflected upon; perhaps a less wildly emotional or murderous version might even be sent. Or it can be burned, ripped up or flushed away, destroying some of the violence of feeling with the paper.

Unsent letters and decision making

Never-to-be sent letters can aid clarification. Having painfully decided to take early retirement due to an untenable work situation, Francesco thought he should write, carefully outlining the situation; he also experimentally drafted a likely reply. He wrote without planning, off the top of his head.

Dear MD

My decision to leave my post was a difficult one. I started in 2000 with high hopes that my department would become the foremost in XXX...

I hope you will view these comments in the spirit in which they are intended: as reflections upon an experience which has not been altogether satisfactory but from which, I hope, something can be learnt. I wish you well in leading XXX towards becoming London's Global Organisation.

Francesco

Dear Francesco

Thank you for your letter which you have clearly put a lot of thought into. I can understand that, from your point of view, things have not gone altogether well. But I am sure you can understand that, in an institution as complex as XXX, there are bound to be clashes of interest which will disappoint some. I'm sorry your experience has not been all you had hoped for but understand you have come to an acceptable arrangement for your retirement with our human resources department.

I will give careful thought to some of the points you have made in the spirit you have made them. I wish you well for your early retirement.

With very best wishes

MD

Francesco

Francesco reread the letters reflectively, and shared them confidentially with two trusted others. The reply, a mere polite dismissal, informed him his letter wouldn't be read if sent. After a while the complete disengagement of the reply made him laugh, realising it was just how the MD would respond. He saw there was no point in sending a letter, that the whole exercise had been a personally developing reflective one. He began to face his early retirement with positive plans and a lighter heart.

SENT LETTERS, NOTES AND POEMS

Writing can enable us to communicate with each other effectively when speech would be difficult or even impossible. This is because I can be privately alone when writing, and recipients need not have me in front of them when reading. This space and solitude allows for reflection, which can be kind and wise. Writers can prepare missives thoughtfully, drafting and redrafting as wanted and needed. Readers have the preparation of slitting an envelope and unfolding the paper, or they need not open and read a letter or email immediately. They can take time before responding.

Sent letters and terminal illness

A young mother dying of cancer wrote to her two daughters in her last days. Too poorly to write, she dictated and signed, and they were delivered after her death. Letters of love, care and loss, they also expressed hope for their future.

She also wrote to her husband before this. Having got the hang of the power of letter writing by writing a lengthy letter to her cancer, she realised it could be used to communicate to real people things she couldn't bring herself to utter. When she could still use her hands she wrote: 'Dear M-, I know I am in terrible pain, and my body isn't like it was. But I would still like a cuddle, please. All my love, J-'. She got her cuddles. But her husband told me afterwards, tearfully, that he hadn't realised he could have written back to her. There were things he would have liked to have said, but also couldn't bring himself to voice. He learned too late, very sadly, the full extent of what letter writing can offer.

Sent letters and relationship healing

A mother and teenage daughter reached a point of being unable to communicate with each other, a situation probably familiar to many parents of girls. They overcame it by writing notes to each other and leaving them in the kitchen for the other to find. Some of these notes were practical, such as 'out at a disco tonight, back at 11pm'. Some of them were entreating, 'PLEASE tidy your room!', and some touching, 'I do love you really'.

> I wrote a piece for publication about caring for my mother through dementia, and had to get my sister's permission, which I knew would be difficult. As children we were very close; as adults we have grown apart, and the writing exposed our differences. In an intense email exchange we each stated our case, point by point. I redrafted with close attention to her responses and really began to want to reflect her particular voice, her thinking; it made for better writing. She thanked me, and we ended up collaborating on finer details. She still pointed out she did not share my sentiments and wanted to distance herself from my writing. Surprisingly the e-mail communication bridged a rift, where talking couldn't. We worked through something together through the power of writing.
>
> *Monica Suswin*

An elderly couple, who had worked as a business partnership and therefore had had a history of being together much of the time, found on retirement that silences grew and spread within their relationship. The husband closed the gap by writing notes, written on scraps and envelope backs, left on the dining table. These were often angry, vituperative and unprintable; he also wrote the opposite, such as 'I love you and want you to have everything in the world you want. XXX'. Here is another example, this time from youth:

> For a few months in the summer when we were sixteen, my best friend and I wrote letters to each other. In June 1973 I wrote in my journal: 'It may sound silly, as we see each other almost every day; but we decided that talk is a bit inhibiting and we can say things we really

mean in letters. I believe these letters will echo a new lease of life in our friendship.' My journal charts the anticipation before each letter, both given and received. This brief correspondence seems to have been romantic without the romance. Perhaps that summer of letters helped us struggle through to a deeper understanding, helped us develop into the close adult friends we became, until I was with him when he died eighteen years later. If those overblown soul-searching letters helped us achieve that, I'm grateful to them, even though, like Clifford, their words are now part of the air.

Robert Hamberger

In the Netherlands such note-writing communication is formalised on a single day of the year.

Personal Poems

The evening of SINTERKLAAS is an old Dutch tradition. We celebrate the Saint's birthday on the 5th or 6th December. Young children put their shoes under the chimney to receive presents in them as Sinterklaas rides on the roofs on his white horse. Older children and adults who do not believe in Sinterklaas anymore have their special feast. Presents are exchanged with poems and so-called *surprises*: an opportunity to tease loved ones with stupid or funny things they have done, or with their more general character traits and behaviour. Your poem expresses your thoughts anonymously because all poems are signed by Sinterklaas, though author's styles are immediately recognized in families. I once fooled mine by making a very mean poem about myself, and I could see everyone thinking: this is going too far, who wrote this?

Sinterklaas is perhaps a psychologically very healthy tradition because in a gentle way people who live together tell each other the truth and hold a mirror. Because the idea is to laugh a lot during the evening, one is enabled to 'get it out' but at the same tell each other that you accept and love one another. Obviously the poems tell something about the creativity and the personality of the author. Those who are not very good at poetry concentrate on '*surprises*': a sort of practical joke-present. Some create wonderful things with *papier mache* or other techniques; others use simple symbolic presents. It requires quite a lot of preparation, if you take it seriously. But half of the fun is the secrecy and atmosphere of anticipation: giggling, huge parcels carried through the house, threats – 'I will get you with Sinterklaas'.

Inez de Beaufort

Care over emails

Problematic emails can initially be written as unsent letters: it's too easy to type quickly and click *send*. A British professional support and disciplinary organisation asks staff, including directors, as a matter of course to write and save key emails overnight, to be reread, reflected upon and redrafted if necessary before sending the next day. Writing them in the normal computer writing programme (e.g. Word), saving and then copying and pasting into an email the next day, can help create positive distance.

Letters are a form of dialogue. Communication can be just as enlightening when written in a similar way to a play. Chapter 9 looks at the explorative and expressive power of written dialogues.

WRITE!

1. Begin every session by writing for *six minutes* with no given subject. Allow the hand to follow the flow of whatever appears on the page: you will find subjects to write about appear on their own: if they don't, then describe something about your surroundings, or that you feel.

2. Think of a time in your childhood which you've always remembered but perhaps are not terribly clear why.

   a. Write a letter to yourself from the child you were then, telling you all about it, including lots of details. Write it in the language that child might use.

   b. Write a letter back to that child-you. Ask the child several questions about the story.

   c. Write the child's responses to the questions.

3. Think of a troublesome part of yourself (such as your stomach if you suffer from persistent indigestion).

    a. Write a letter to this troublesome part of yourself. Ask it any questions you feel are pertinent.

    b. Write back as if from that part of your body, answering the questions, and telling why you cause trouble.

4. Write a letter to yourself in the future.

    a. Tell this self about your life now: its successes, joys and difficulties.

    b. Write the reply telling your present self about how it is in the future. Allow this future self to give advice to your present self.

5. a. Write a letter to Santa.

    b. Write Santa's reply.

6. Reread all your writing reflectively and generously to yourself. Allow any further thoughts to surface and add them in, or alter your writing in any way which seems right. Remember you can always alter again and re-alter at any time. There might be interesting connections between the *Six Minute Write* and another piece.

CHAPTER 9

Conversation with Myself

'I'm in two minds about this' and 'I can't make up my mind' are common experiences. Yet, we are often in far more than 'two minds' about something: once a problematic situation is reflected upon in depth, a range of possibilities generally surfaces. One of these is often a much better way forward than the two possibilities we felt stuck with before; the reason for the stuckness was that neither original strategy was right.

Each of us has wells of wisdom and understanding in our complex beings. Much of this is often untapped, because in our culture we tend to feel a need to be consistent, and so have not found strategies for gaining value from diverse and often wonderful elements of our characters. Being 'single minded' is seen as a positive attribute; a good way towards such consistency is by experiencing and exploring the complexity first. In a similar way, a researcher struggles to acquire as wide a range of data as possible, before examining it to reach her conclusions.

A positive way out of a seemingly intractable dilemma is literally to 'make up' our minds, in the same way as we make up, or create, a story. Stories contain conversations or dialogues between people. Writing such dialogues between the dynamic different elements of ourselves can enhance awareness of this multiplicity and can be an effective way to help 'make up' our minds.

A dialogue, or conversation, with the self can be an enlightening route to helping us find our wiser selves, and to face our less wise elements positively. A classic way of seeing an internal dialogue is between *head* and *heart*. It can be set out rather like a playscript, or more like a story as Sue has here.

My head urges me to plan, to sequence, to meet aims and objectives, to analyse and critically evaluate, to fit a model, to meet criteria, to meet academic standards, to please others – teachers, professionals, writers, professors, experts, parents. To prove myself, to gain affirmation, credibility, status, acclaim, respect, validation, fame?

My heart is having none of it. My heart rebels and resists all attempts to create an intellectual masterpiece. My heart screams and pounds so loudly to STOP playing the game. 'What an immensely boring story that would be' winces Heart.

NO!! My head argues, trying desperately to quell and suppress. 'You must write a paper', 'Research and write a thesis', ' You need to do a doctorate.'

STOP!! Says Heart. No more! 'Follow ME. I will guide you and show you the way. Please do not be a sheep, a follower, a lemming. Stand tall and be yourself. Find your voice. Speak your truth. You have something worth saying, so believe in yourself. Have courage, and SAY IT'.

OK, I am listening, I say. I trust you, and believe in you, so I give you my pen. Go ahead and tell the tale. Your tale. Your truth. YOUR STORY. Tell it Sue. Just for you. For yourself.

Sue McDonald

There are many other aspects of ourselves we can have conversations with. There are many more personal qualities to explore and harness, or struggle with, in writing. A really close friend might astonish by seeming to become a different person in a setting we've never seen them in before: wiser perhaps, more jovial, or quieter and more circumspect. I have amazed myself by finding fortitude or patience I did not previously know I had, when faced with a demanding situation. And we all have private conversations with ourselves, and habits, fears, memories we never tell anyone about, often even trying to hide them from ourselves. The more we struggle not to be aware of such anxieties or unwelcome wishes, the more they will not go away, often destructively in the middle of the night.

WHY DIALOGUE?

This chapter shows how we can pay constructive attention to more of our facets. Written conversations, as if with different elements of ourselves or with people we can't talk to in reality, can illuminate. Inventing characters to speak, a bit like a play, can help us hear some of the quieter more divergent elements of ourselves, and to recognise dominant facets. Similar to unsent letter writing, these conversations are written quickly and dynamically.

They use methods borrowed from play and fiction writing, though they are not intended to be acted or spoken. Najwa lost her only child, her son, and wrote in poetry form:

> With Haas gone, I had to find a way to stay connected with him. I imagined talking to him. It felt real and it was comforting.
>
> **Come fly with me**, mom
> We'll go places you have never seen
> I'll show you sites of which you only dreamed
> You'll be free like a breeze, like me
> Wandering in the cosmos
> with love and peace.
>
> **I love to fly with you**, son
> But I'm sorry my wings are not working
> Since my heart was broken
> when you left suddenly to the other side
> Can I fly if I set my wings aside?
>
> **Open your arms** and let go of the past
> Lift yourself smoothly off to the skies
> Keep your heart calm and your eyes towards the stars
> Look up for me, I'll be in sight
> Hold my hand tight and together we zoom into the light
> Where love and peace reside
> You'll fly.
> Yes, you'll fly.
> When you let go, when you let me go
> You'll fly.
>
> *Najwa Mounla, Haas's mom*

Philosophers and young children question and question, trying to work out for themselves what they think and believe about such as faith, justice, truth, honesty, integrity, openness, fairness, non-discrimination and other fundamental values. Life constantly throws us dilemmas where we are not clear what is right and wrong.

One of the first philosophers invented dialogues as a brilliant way of trying to understand what people thought and believed. Plato wrote many stories about his teacher Socrates, a practical wise Athenian. These stories often concern an evening of good food, wine, a floor show, and then – most important – discussion written in dialogue form. The accounts are entertaining and fascinating over two thousand years later, because Socrates helped people work out what they thought by having lengthy, well-illustrated arguments. Socrates was said to be like a midwife to his students' intellect, knowledge and imagination: setting it free from the narrowness of the birth-canal, and constraints of the womb.

Most of us will never achieve the brilliance and aplomb of Socrates. His method of reflecting using written dialogues can be copied, however. Plato tells us Socrates never gave his students answers, because he didn't know the answers himself. He countered their queries, asked questions, led them to face areas they needed to examine and reflect upon – coming up with their own answers.

Discussions can be written between myself and a wise invented character a bit like Socrates (who might be female). This character (it's useful to find out their name) will never TELL you what you think or believe, but will keep asking questions and putting points until you are clearer.

SELF: I HATE teaching. How did I ever come to make such a wrong decision? How can I get out of it now?

RAFI: 1. steady money. 2. keeps you busy – less time to worry about Ted. What's wrong with it?

SELF: The kids all talk at once and can't keep still. I HATE stopping them as I know that's what children do – naturally – schools are unnatural. I end up shouting.

RAFI: What would you rather do?

SELF: Oh I don't know! I can't go back to administration – I was happy but HATED being told what to do all the time!

RAFI: Lots of HATE! What do you love?

SELF: Children! Helping people learn! Schools aren't for learning but controlling though.

RAFI: There's lots of teaching which isn't classroom – have you thought about it?

This dialogue went on and on, written on several occasions. *Rafi* required the woman to make a wide range of lists weighing up different elements of her life, to help her decide what to do. Eventually she became a learning support teacher: working with one child at a time.

WHERE DO CHARACTERS COME FROM?

Characters powerfully dialogue their way through a book or play's plot. They seem to speak and think like real people, and we as audience are able to empathise with them, and learn or expand our awareness from how they cope with events and relate to each other.

Character interchanges only *seem* to be lifelike. More is included than in real speech, which tends to be bitty and disjointed: people butt in and talk across each other. Shakespeare does this most spectacularly. Possibly Britain's greatest playwright, he put lengthy complex clever speeches in the mouths of the very young lovers Romeo and Juliet, for example; in real life they would have done little more than grunt and utter other teenage inarticulacies.

Key writing helps us borrow novelists' or playwrights' flexible methods. A non-writers' enduring fantasy is that writers re-create real people they know directly onto the page. That would be impossible, though of course elements of friends, family, colleagues and foes contribute to fictional character development. We can all re-create our child self, and powerful others: the head-teacher who told me I was useless at everything except making mischief; my parents' and siblings' voices in different ways; and some strong helpers like Socrates. Here is Caleb Lambert:

> **CHILD ME**: OK, Mr Policeman, You feel that dwelling on my work problems before I went into hospital is unhelpful. Why? What's the problem?

> **POLICEMAN**: Your time in hospital marks a break and your life now marks a new chapter. You need to be looking forward not back. Life's full of new possibilities. You don't want to be dwelling on old grievances and hurts.

> **CHILD ME**: But maybe I can't move on without coming to terms with what's happened in the past. I want some space to indulge my hurts.

POLICEMAN: If you must, but the attraction will soon wear thin. There's far more interesting and enjoyable things you could be doing.

CHILD ME: Such as?

POLICEMAN: Well… Meeting new challenges. Writing the next chapter of your story which has changed course so dramatically.

CHILD ME: But maybe the way into the future is through the past? Maybe the key lies in unlocking the richness of your past, not turning the page and pretending nothing has gone before. I just want to be left to play and see what happens.

POLICEMAN: (momentarily wrongfooted) All right. Go ahead. Play. See where it gets you…

Caleb Lambert

DIALOGUES WITH THE INNER CHILD

Characters to talk to can be invented or imagined as parts of the self. Everyone grows up and away from childish hopes and fears, hatreds and desires. For many, all these can happily be consigned to a mental box labelled *childish memories*. But for some, that child inside still feels lost, lonely and abandoned, still longs for unattainable, but perfectly reasonable goodies of life. The harder such a person tries to jam the lid on that memory box, the more it pops off when least wanted. In this extract, Francesca discovered how she was neglecting her inner child:

My friend suggested the only way to get through my siblings coming to my daughter's 21st birthday was to find out what my inner child was feeling. I wrote this in my journal:

ME: I don't want to do this, but I will. What am I afraid of? What are you feeling little Fran?

LITTLE FRAN: I feel abandoned. Like I really can't trust you because you aren't taking very good care of me. You keep not feeding me properly, you don't listen when I am crying and now you are going to take me to that horrible place again. I HATE THEM – I DON'T WANT TO BE MADE TO SEE THEM AGAIN – THEY HURT

ME – ALL OF THEM HURT ME. I THOUGHT WE WERE SAFE AND AWAY FROM ALL OF IT. I FEEL REALLY REALLY SICK LIKE I COULD END UP IN HOSPITAL – YOU WILL KILL ME IF YOU DON'T LISTEN. YOU CAN DO ANYTHING YOU WANT, GO ANYWHWERE YOU WANT AS LONG AS YOU TAKE CARE OF ME, FEED ME, LOOK AFTER ME PROPERLY. THEN YOU CAN DO THIS. Please.

ME: I feel your anger and that is why I experience you as the enemy. I do starve and neglect you and I am so sorry.

After this dialogue I really became aware of getting enough food, good food, 3 times a day. And enough sleep and good personal grooming. For that whole week I was still afraid, but the terror subsided. When my 3 sisters came they ran up an alcohol bill of £200 which they didn't pay for and I felt their hostility – I felt SAFE AND SOBER! My daughter enjoyed her party and I learnt that I really can do anything if I take care of that little girl first.

Francesca Creffield

Simon struggled with depression and anxiety which seemed to have no cause. He discovered his inner child, calling him Brian: giving him a name was really helpful. It took several writing attempts before little Brian started tentatively to say what had hurt him so badly.

Remembering fragments of his past, although painful, was helpful: forgetting them had only created problems. He realised how much going away to boarding school aged seven had affected him. There had been no-one to turn to about terrifying maths, having to eat disgusting food and drink tepid milk. Brian was able to remind Simon of the aching loneliness of going to bed alone at this young age, and then coming home for the holidays to find his beloved young dog had been put down.

Simon slowly linked present anxiety with past pain. He became tearfully unhappy on an overseas business trip, as if he were never coming home; he learned that going away alone, and taking work with him, felt like going back to school. He discovered that his annual autumn depression was linked to the end of the long school summer holidays.

When Simon was writing one day, another boy started answering, a happy child. This child – Jumping Jim – encouraged Simon to turn melancholy thoughts inside out, to look outwards at the beauty and life around him, and enjoy it; to dance into difficult situations optimistically rather than feeling leaden and fearful. Simon learned, once he had heard Bruised Brian's miserable accounts, always then to turn to Jim and hear his joyful ones, and to make future plans with him. He learned how to balance opposing childlike ways of feeling within him.

Erika Mansnerus, a postdoctoral research fellow, is writing her first book. To help her face the likelihood of a higher profile that this publication and an academic career might bring her, she explored her feelings by imagining a dialogue with a child.

> I'm afraid of success, the little boy said. If I run as fast as I can, nobody will like me. If I'm good at school, nobody will be my friend. I looked at him. His blue eyes were full of honesty and openness, but also fear. I looked at him silently. This was not a moment to repeat the empty sentences of well-wishing. No, his fear was deeper and more concrete to be comforted with flat sentences, echoing emptiness in the air.
>
> I had known him only since September. We met by a green, leafy stream in Wales. I was there on my daily walk and he was fishing and wandering around. Like an explorer in a new world. I looked at him there were no words between us and no need for words either.
>
> Can you hear me? he asked in a demanding tone. I am lonely as I am and the least I want is to be bullied. He carried on with exhausting energy. Look, I know a girl in the other class and she is the best. Always there, homework done, and she is really lonely. I listened with sadness in my heart. How difficult it is for us to be brave in what we are. I heard his pain of loneliness and knew that he had to make a difficult choice.
>
> Have you thought of the successful ones? I asked. Have you thought of your heroes? They have a lonely path but eventually they become popular. The boy was listening intensively. Look at the people who run fastest, jump highest and write the best stories: they create the best out of their lives by facing the lonely paths. The boy's eyes sparkled, as if he'd seen something I didn't.
>
> *By writing this story, I gave words to my deeper fears about success. Will I be accepted if I explore the world freely among the best? The wise tone*

of the author points to the key question: I am facing the boy's choice. And that choice will lead to lonely paths, but also towards a more contented and satisfied way of being who I am.

Erika Mansnerus

DIALOGUES WITH THE INNER ADULT

Many cultures have imagined we each have an opposite personality, called such as *alter ego*, *doppelganger*. An introverted quiet woman was perpetually anxious when asked to do things, felt she made a muddle of them, and constantly blamed herself for things going wrong. She invented a strong capable and sensible character called Diana. Whenever she worried about a piece of work or family event she discussed it with Diana, asking for advice. Dear Diana never failed her: always writing back in a firm confident hand listing the order of things which should be done, and telling her everything would be OK. And even if it didn't go perfectly she said: 'well nobody's going to die are they?' The woman found an old photograph amongst family papers of an unknown ancestor in a long crinolined frock. Deciding it was Diana, she found a simple frame and kept her visibly on her desk. She continued to write dialogues regularly, but Diana's face smiling firmly at her, the direct look in her eyes, always made her back straighten and enabled her to pick up the phone decisively, write a strong email or make sensible workable plans.

One man discusses his life with Juggler Josh. A professional trainer and coach, he needs to be constantly inventive, flexible and imaginative, yet sensitive and aware of others' needs, moods and wants. Inevitably sometimes exhausted or run out of initiative, he turns in his journal to Juggler Josh: generally to be relied upon to provide support, advice and fresh energetic ideas. Once, though, Juggler Josh said he had nothing to give: it was time to take a rest or he'd get burnt out. It was wise advice: after a refreshing holiday he could continue: reinvigorated, and grateful to his internal partner.

Here is Monica again.

I am dealing with a lot of different types of feeling through this writing. The voices take on their own imaginative life and I then become the observer of my own inner drama. It is theatre in the unfolding: the writing arriving with its own agenda.

How do I know this writing is helpful? It makes me feel good. And the writing adopts something of what the child wants when things go wrong. They want to run to Mummy and tell her all about it. It helps me take charge of my inner emotional life in an adult way.

Why do we need our inner Mummies? The mothering part of myself helps the hurt part – through the act of writing. Each of us only has one real mother, but we can be nurturing to ourselves without being over-caring, over-protective or over-solicitous, just as good-enough mothering allows separation and independence.

Monica Suswin

Everyone can discover their own inner characters through reflection. Francesca found so many to talk to that she had to imagine them all on a bus. It felt good at the end of a writing session to shut and lock the bus door, keeping them all in safely and in communication with each other. I would like to suggest there are two further inner characters to communicate with: mentor and personality terrorist. Chapter 10 gives many ways of strengthening the former, so the latter becomes less destructively dominant.

WRITE!

1. Begin every session by writing for *six minutes* with no given subject. Allow the hand to follow the flow of whatever appears on the page: you will find subjects to write about appear on their own: if they don't, then describe something about your surroundings, or that you feel.

2. In the middle of your forehead you have a point where your all-perceiving eye might be: your eye of insight. I call this the *Sky Eye*. Ask your own *Sky Eye* questions like this:

   • What can you see?

   • How is it different from what my normal eyes can see?

   • Please tell me your perspective on my current problem (state your problem).

   Write *Sky Eye*'s response, and continue the dialogue. You might like to do this briefly and regularly, in a way similar to the *Six Minute Write*: a kind of 'checking in' process.

3. Seeing things from the other person's point of view, where possible. Think of a person who's made your life difficult in some way.

   a. Write an account, a narrative of a really tough time with them.

   b. Now go back over the narrative and underline all the important moments.

   What was the difficult person thinking then? How did she/he experience the situation? See if you can write just what they were thinking at those moments, a bit like cartoon thought bubbles.

   c. Turn it into a dialogue with you responding to their every thought.

4. Write describing an important place which you use regularly, such as office, kitchen, classroom, or consulting room.

   a. Describe yourself coming into it in the morning, every little thing you do. Write as if observing yourself; call yourself 'you'.

   b. Write a response from the point of view of a colleague or friend you like and admire, describing their own office, kitchen, classroom or consulting room, coming in first thing in the morning and what they do (they call themselves 'I').

   c. Write a dialogue with both yourself and your friend or colleague, asking if there's any way you could alter your room or space to make you happier or more effective in it.

5. Reread reflectively, being generous to yourself. Make any alterations which seem useful, and share the writing with a trusted other, if that feels good.

CHAPTER 10

Mentors and Terrorists

We all have a powerful wise side of our selves. Sometimes it's hard to hear it clearly, let alone allow it to support us. We all also have self-destructive inner forces which are stronger in some than others. Valuing our diverse array of strengths, as well as attending properly to weaknesses, can help empower the former and go some way to developing positive strategies against the latter. This chapter offers playful and satisfying methods.

Mentor was originally a goddess in disguise, on earth to help Odysseus' young son search for his father who'd been lost at sea for ten years. Mentor's wisdom and judicial powers enabled a tangled mess of events to be sorted out, at least according to Homer's Odyssey over two thousand years ago. We can't all call on the help of a goddess, but can each find within ourselves a strong wise character to offer advice and support on any issue from the most mundane to the life-changing. A way of making contact with this character, this inner life-coach or mentor, is to write letters or dialogues.

Inside each of us is also a self-destructive force. I call this nagging, whining, bullying element the inner terrorist, or critic. Many people think this negative voice is just themselves, not realising it can be counteracted and efforts made to banish it. Feeling the inner terrorist is their real self is why many find journal writing deeply unsatisfying. They get stuck with the voice of this terrorist; it makes them even more depressed and they don't know how to shake it off. *Key* writing has powerful processes to counteract such destructive forces.

THE INTERNAL LIFE-COACH

A family doctor (GP) called her newly discovered inner life-coach Aurora, meaning dawn.

Dear Aurora

I suppose the greatest joy I have in writing to you is that I can never be wrong in what I say or ask of you.

You never judge or criticise, but always offer constructive guidance, another perspective, or challenge me to stretch myself, open my mind or think again.

You always reply to my contacts so honestly and helpfully, and I look forward with excitement to your comments.

You are immune to the concrete things of the world like power cuts or postal strikes – your message will always reach me, wherever I am, whatever I am doing, whatever I ask of you.

I trust you wholly and know you will guide me wisely and lovingly.

You let me say anything don't you – and in doing so, feelings crystallise and troubles resolve themselves.

What matters most is that I know you are there for ME – always and forever.

Thank you.

Lucy Henshall

Any issue or problem can be given to the internal mentor in writing; I do it all the time in my journal. Sometimes when particularly stuck, I realise it's because I've forgotten to ask my journal.

People sometimes ask me 'should I do this or that?' 'Ask your writing!' I say. Once opened out in writing, several options generally come to light. It can seem like magic: but of course it's not. When things weigh heavy, it's often hard to see beyond them: thinking can go round and around in increasingly useless repetitive circles. Writing can leap over the walls of such stifling prisons. To use my original image: it gives us the key to the dark cell's door. Caleb was extremely ill and used writing to help him find strength for the ordeals he was undergoing:

'So who are you?'

'I'm your Spiritual Father.'

'So what are you saying to me?'

'I actually think you've coped pretty well with what's been a terribly difficult time – completely outside your previous experience. Nothing has really prepared you for it. You have learnt to try and live with the situation in which you find yourself, not rail against it futilely or self-pityingly bemoan your fate (and you can certainly be excused for doing that occasionally). You will seek to justify our existence by what you do though. That's what's been frustrating and upsetting you recently. You need to realise there are times to be "done to", times when being is more important, times when what you are is more important.'

'And what am I?'

'Frightened frustrated, bemused. Brave, resilient, coping (just!). Not defeated (if occasionally bowled over). A loving husband and caring father. A loyal friend. A seeker after understanding and truth, even if those things often seem to baffle and elude you.'

'Crikey…'

'You shouldn't be embarrassed. There's lots of other nice things I could say about you. But because you're not doing much at present, your self-esteem is low, you feel lacking in self-worth. Unjustified… If there's one piece of advice I'd give you, it's to "listen" to allow yourself to see things from a different perspective to the goal-driven, activity-led angle that you're used to. You may find a shape or purpose (a "justification") to what's going on in your life that you had no idea existed – that the role you have to play, the contribution you are able to make is already present and taking shape. Learn to contemplate if life is forcing you to sit still…'

'So much to unlearn…'

'No. Re-learn. Or just learn. All part of being human. It doesn't stop just because you're in your late forties.'

'"Teach us to sit still." I don't feel I've a great deal of option.'

'So go with it. It won't be forever.'

Caleb Lambert

The internal life-coach can help solve problems, alleviate anxieties and sense of inadequacy or failure. This mentor is invaluable when planning or needing a confidence boost before an event, or debriefing or feedback after a meeting, or any other work, social or family occasion. A mother wrote many anxious journal entries, dealing with fears about parenting her young son. Her mentor speaks here from her journal.

> I'm a mother. I'm there, sticking plaster and food at the ready, to bandage and comfort. I try to stand back, to be a friend and a listener now, to give him wings. But he's not ready to fly, so I hover around, never going too far from the nest. I'm a taxi driver, cook and, if he needs me, a counsellor. I'm a social secretary and with all this I try to enable him to learn and become independent. My apron strings are very loose now but not quite ready to break. I'm not a flowery domesticated, *Little House on the Prairie* Mum. But I'm OK.
>
> *Fiona Friend*

Many things happen around us which go unnoticed because we're focussed in a different direction. All this unnoticed stuff is stored in our minds, however: generally never known about, even less used. Writing can give the key to some of this storehouse of information. So-called mind-readers tune their senses to pick up as much as possible of the information other people give unintentionally about their thoughts and feelings. They use these clues to make it seem they know what people are thinking.

Writers make mind-readers of themselves. Writing can help us become more aware of what's going on around us and in our own heads: what we know and understand without realising it. We habitually live our lives only noticing a narrow range of information. The storehouses in our minds remain locked and bolted, and relationships – work, social or family – suffer.

A probably even more ancient guide than the disguised goddess, Mentor, was the archangel Raphael. He pretends to be a servant to help a lad called Tobit go on a long journey to reclaim his father's treasure (the Book of Tobit in the *Apocrypha*). Even more importantly Raphael helps Tobit find medicine to cure his father's blindness. We can think of the treasure as an image for happiness, and the medicine as curing not physical blindness but enabling philosophical and spiritual insight. Raphael proved himself to be as powerful a teacher and guide as Mentor. Here is a father in conversation with his internal mentor:

A father's dialogue

Me

Please tell me what I really said to Tom. It was so awful I got so angry. PLEASE – what did Tom say – and – think?

Mentor

Now you're cool, look back, remember Tom's face, voice, remember how he spoke. I think Tom was really really upset. He's much younger than you. And you have all the power. I think he's really worried, and – well – frightened. What do you think he went and did?

Me

Oh no, he went up to his room to cry didn't he? Or the nearest he'd get to crying. I thought he was angry too! He's only a boy and I'm a powerful man… Have I alienated him completely? I know – I'll make sure I'm there when he comes home tomorrow – get off work early – surprise him – ask him to come to the park with the football, or if I can do his homework with him. Both perhaps! Thank you!

You can have your own Mentor or Raphael available 24 hours a day, every day of the year, all your life.

THE PERSONALITY TERRORIST

Writing can cope with, or counteract, internalised critical forces. Adults, and particularly children, are surrounded by instructions: what to do, how to do it, with whom, when and where; all these often with no explanation of why. These know-alls (parents, bosses, tutors, teachers, partners, husbands, wives…) instruct, advise and generally know better. Yet we hold authority over our own adult lives and decisions. In losing it we lose self-respect, self-worth and ability, and love of work for its own sake. Writing offers a way of taking whole-hearted responsibility, resisting mental negative forces, putting positive ones in their place.

Must, should, ought, shouldn't and *CAN'T* can be seen as the terrorist's or critic's wagging finger. Everyone has internalised a bullying voice to some extent, perhaps starting with a parent or teacher. It nags inside the mind, saying we're no good, won't and can't succeed. We begin to believe we are inadequate personally, socially or professionally, stupid, inarticulate, ugly, fat, gauche. It then seems easier and better not to try: to hide in a corner at the party, remain silent at the meeting, not go for the big new job, carry on drinking far too much alcohol, wear the cover-all shapeless tent dress, not expose flab in the gym, and so on and on.

One of the secrets is to distinguish the voice of the destructive critic as soon as it starts: it is so insistent and clever it sneaks under our defences. We all have a stronger voice in us which can say: *I WON'T listen to you! I WILL listen to my wiser internal guides!* Many mistake their inner critic for themselves. Separating it off and giving it recognisable characteristics makes it possible to tackle. Poet Ted Hughes reckoned he had to 'outwit his own inner police system, which told him what is permissible, what is possible, what is "him"' (1982, p.7). The policemen tried to instruct him how he should be. The novelist Virginia Woolf had a domestic angel trying to mould her into the Victorian ideal of the socially acceptable woman.

> The Angel in the House…excelled in the difficult arts of family life. She sacrificed herself daily…so constituted that she never had a mind or wish of her own, but preferred to sympathise always with the minds and wishes of others… The shadow of her wings fell on my page…directly I took my pen in my hand…she slipped behind me and…made as if to guide my pen… I turned upon her and caught her by the throat. I did my best to kill her. She would have plucked the heart out of my writing… It is far harder to kill a phantom than a reality. She was always creeping back when I thought I had despatched her.
>
> *Virginia Woolf (1979[1931], p.60)*

Hughes and Woolf were brilliant writers, but neither biddable nor socially conformist: they tackled their destructive inner critics for the sake of their work. They can be models for us: in the pursuit of being true to ourselves we can locate our own inner terrorist, and destroy or work out strategies to outwit it. Giving it metaphorical form (policeman, cloying domestic angel, black parrot) helps put flesh on its bones.

'It is far harder to kill a phantom than a reality.' Yes, but writing gives communication with this phantom: far more powerful than trying to silence and destroy a formless nagging in the mind. Here is part of Dorothy Nimmo's powerful poem about her experience:

Black Parrot

Kill the black parrot. Choke the sodding bird,
it never said a kind thing or a true word
or if it did that wasn't what I heard.

I only heard its squawking in my ear
things no-one in their right mind wants to hear
that made me cold with shame and white with fear.

Behave yourself. Control yourself. You know
You don't think that, you only think you do.
You can't just please yourself. I told you so...

Dorothy Nimmo (1993, p.7)

One of my internal critics is Sensible Susan. Lips pursed tightly against any softness or care, hair scragged back to go with her unremittingly sensible clothes, she frowns critically, instructing me to pull myself together and get on with it instead of mooning about. There's no mending the fact I'm plain, stupid, untidy, disorganised, inarticulate in conversation, and not good at anything much. Many times I've wished I could click my fingers for Mary Poppins to sail through the window with her umbrella wings instead. I do my best by writing as many of Sensible Susan's poisoned words as I can so they can be trapped safely between the covers of my journal. Then Raphael, or one of the others, can counteract her: writing wise constructive words.

Winston Churchill (and eighteenth-century Samuel Johnson) was famously tormented by a 'black dog'. A 'black dog on your back', an old expression, was sometimes perceived as the devil: an apt image for the internal critic. Internal Critics or Personality Terrorists dog many people. Never far away with their whining or hectoring voices, they are a frequent cause of depression, lack of self-confidence and self-esteem. Discovering the voice of the wise Internal Mentor and making space to listen to it clearly, creates the strength to disable any internal terrorist. Jane C's approach was to write an acrostic:

SOAP
Slay the inner critic
Over his dead body
Attack his heart
Paint victory on your paper

Jane Calne

Such conversations put us in touch with ourselves. Chapter 11 uncovers how dreams are a powerhouse of characters to converse with. Mental, spiritual, imaginative, night-dream and day-dream lives are richer than most people ever realise or use. Once aware of that wealth of knowledge, experience, ability to understand, discuss, describe, feel and intuit we have the power to take far greater control of our lives.

WRITE!

1. Begin every session by writing for *six minutes* with no given subject. Allow the hand to follow the flow of whatever appears on the page: you will find subjects to write about appear on their own: if they don't, then describe something about your surroundings, or that you feel.

2. Make a list, writing a phrase or sentence for each entry. If your Internal Mentor were one of these, what or who would they be?

   • an animal

   • a plant of any sort

   • a food or drink

   • a relative or someone else from your past

   • make up your own categories.

   Describe she/he/it in more detail, using ideas from what you've just written.

3. Make up the kindest most helpful knowledgeable person or being you can imagine. Give her/him/it a name. This only really works if you invent someone or something, or use an off-the-peg one like Angel Raphael or the Goddess Athene.

   a. Write this being a letter asking for advice or help with a specific problem or issue.

   b. Write the reply, which might be lengthy. Continue the dialogue or letters if you wish. This doesn't always work the first time; if so, just leave it for a while and have a go another time.

4. Make a list, writing a phrase or sentence for each entry.

    a. If your Internal Terrorist or Critic were one of these, what would they be?

    *   an insect

    *   a sci-fi or fantasy creature (invent one, but think of Tolkein, Harry Potter, Star Wars, etc.)

    *   a relative or someone else from your past

    *   a cleaning material or equipment

    *   make up your own categories.

    b. How does it:

    *   walk and move?

    *   communicate with you?

    *   live with you (think of the parrot on the shoulder, dog on the back)?

    *   attack you, and when?

    *   remind you of someone?

    *   make its presence felt normally?

    c. Write a dialogue or set of letters to and from this aspect of yourself.

5. List critical things you say to yourself in your mind.

    a. Make the list as long as you can: up to 20 if possible (50 even better). Try to be honest, remembering NO-ONE else need ever read this. If you get stuck, think of activities you find difficult (formal family occasion, demanding work presentation, letter or other piece of writing). And don't be afraid to repeat yourself as often as you like. The items you repeat are the vital ones. Think specifically of what you find difficult: what are the words that come with lack of confidence, fear or anxiety?

    b. List all the things you tell yourself you *should, ought, must do.*
    All these are probably spoken in the voice of your internal personality saboteur or critic.

c. Pick one from your lists. Write in a free-flow *Six Minute Write* way about it; this might be:

- the critical voice given full reign to shout and rant onto the page: safely now because you know you are learning to be proof against its bullying

- a pouring out of thoughts and feelings in a reflective, possibly rather disorganised way

- an account of an event: include as many details as occur to you, as fully as you can.

Imagine your Critic speaking in the voice of whatever you described in response to 3. If it doesn't work, have another go at depicting it (as in 3 above).

6. Write a dialogue (see Chapter 9) between your Internal Mentor and your Internal Terrorist or Critic. Give them full rein to say what they both feel and think of each other and you.

7. You don't have to read your writing in response to 3 and 4 if you don't want to. You could even destroy it if that felt good. If you do reread, do it with attention, taking note of anything which surprises you or you feel needs developing. Be gentle with yourself. Make sure you ALWAYS end with the voice of the Internal Mentor.

CHAPTER 11

Dreams

WHY DREAMS ARE IMPORTANT

Dreams can offer greater access to the mansion of knowledge, experience and memory. Freud called them the 'Royal Road' to understanding ourselves. This chapter discusses and gives straightforward and enjoyable writing approaches to harness their tremendous power for self-understanding and clarity. Many-roomed, the dream mansion also has walled gardens, spacious summer houses and packed garden sheds. The more explored, the more will be found: the inside much bigger than the outside, like Dr Who's famous Tardis.

Dreams are a rich source of images and stories to play with in writing. They offer wealth, wherever they come from and whatever their significance. Dreams need attention in order to give their gifts. It's too easy to wake up, scramble into thinking about the day ahead or remembering the previous day. Ignored, most of them will simply disappear from consciousness. Courted, re-experienced in writing, and with that writing discussed, dream-life can become an essential part of writing. They might not foretell the future as people once thought, but they do have immense potential to offer insight into more hidden parts of ourselves.

Dreams are an expression of the creative side of us all. Creating fear, anxiety, hope or joy seemingly out of nothing at all, they cannot be controlled, as artistic inspiration beyond control. However clever an analysis or interpretation, there is always another way of looking at a dream. The significance of dream images and stories is open to interpretive explorations by each dreamer and each person who hears the dream recounted; just as artists do not hold the monopoly on knowing what their pictures, sculptures, poems, symphonies, dances signify.

WHAT TO DO WITH A DREAM

Writing can explore and experiment with the richness of dreams: whatever you think of doing will be right for you. Remembering a dream is the first thing. Many say they don't dream, which means they haven't built remembering them into their lives. On waking in the morning remain lying in the same position, as moving can make the dream slip away from consciousness. Stay there reflecting for a few minutes, without trying to wake up further. Then describe or tell the story of the dream in writing.

A single dream image can give much. I dreamed about opening a wooden kitchen cupboard and there being nothing at all in it. It was a very difficult period for me; everything seemed hard and I was struggling to hang onto a sense of proportion and hope. The nursery rhyme from my childhood about Old Mother Hubbard, who had a completely empty cupboard with not even a bone for her dog, came into my mind. What a sense of poverty; this didn't lift my despondent mood at all.

Then I decided to free-write from the image of this emptiness; I dialogued with the cupboard, and crucially with its owner. The writing I wrote then, and worked on, redrafted and reflected upon a great deal, did bring much hope and lightness into my life. All from the seemingly unpromising beginning of a totally empty cupboard.

'Reach up high, onto the high shelf!'
I had to fetch a stepladder, brush my hand
over cobwebby planks; but the whole cupboard
was empty as Mother Hubbard's.

'Try again', you said.
Still nothing.

'You're not looking properly!'
And there it was.

But how could something so infinitesimal
be what I'm looking for?

When I shook it out, I knew what it was:
a pair of wings
just my size.

Gillie Bolton

It's worth working at grasping such seemingly insignificant dream details to work on before they slip away; it doesn't matter how fragmentary they are. I use all sorts of different strategies in my journal.

First I write the story as I remember it IN THE PRESENT TENSE: as if it is happening, rather than last night's dream. Sometimes I think I'm embroidering the dream memory, but that doesn't matter as imagination and dreams come from the same place. I include all the remembered images, though some seem really odd, and quite a lot makes no sense: dreams are not about logical sense.

Sometimes there are people I know in the dream. Dreams, however, pick up people and things to stand for other people or things. I have often dreamt of one of my children when they were little. I don't think the dream was really about them; quite often it's been about my creative child self. Eli dreamt of one of his managers. He felt the dream had nothing to do with the real boss at all, but everything to do with what he stood for: dictatorial bossiness and desire to dominate. I find it helpful to try out different ideas about what I think my dream people might stand for.

I often make a list of all the colours and numbers in a dream, to see if they have significance. I then choose one (once it was the number 4), and do a spider diagram (see Chapter 3) from it. I put the number 4 in the centre of the page, and allowed words and images to fall from my pencil onto the page, clustering as they will. And I did a *Six Minute Write* with the word 'four' at the top of the page. I read through the *Six Minute Write*, and the spider diagram, and chose a word or phrase and wrote from that again. What I learned from developing that insignificant number 4 is still influencing me many years later.

Sometimes I make a list of all the people and things in the dream: for example, table, house, horse, cupboard, money. Sometimes the list contains some very strange and unconnected items. And I write from the perspective of one or more of them, perhaps retelling the story of the dream from their point of view.

One way I look at dreams is to think of every person and every thing as an aspect of me. Of course the house or the baby is also just a house or a baby; everything in a dream has a multiple significance. But for now: I explore thinking that everything on that list is me in some way.

These dream-people and dream-things can then converse. It might seem odd writing a letter beginning *Dear little boy in my dream*, or a dialogue (as if it were a playscript) with the *house in my dream*, but these imaginary conversations tell me an incredible amount. I ask them what they are doing and why, how they can help me, what they have to tell me. They write back to me, telling me things which surprise me, sometimes really really surprise me. I once dreamt I was given two gleaming tiger skins hanging on the wall of an Indian hut; this is what I wrote in my journal:

ME: Tiger skins, why were you given to me? Why would I want a tiger skin, I'd rather a real live tiger! Or perhaps a stuffed toy. It's gruesome.

TIGER SKIN: We are power. You only need one of us. Put me on when you need to feel stronger, particularly in your work. You need the power of 'Tyger, tyger burning bright / In the forests of the night / What immortal hand or eye / Dare frame thy perfect symmetry' (William Blake 1970[1794], p.42).

ME: But I have no right! The skin is yours!

TIGER SKIN: I give you the right to wear my skin. I am a Dream Tiger; so I am free to share my skin as I wish.

ME: Am I brave enough? Am I worthy?

TIGER SKIN: You are afraid of your own power. Everyone is more afraid of their own power than they are of their own weakness. Wear my skin and step into your own power!

ME: And what about the second skin?

TIGER SKIN: You will find out.

That tiger skin gave me the confidence I needed to give the big lecture which was looming. I hate lecturing, being a writer and doer rather than talker. I've worn the tiger skin many times since (nobody else can see it). And the other skin? That's the story of the person I gave it to: she found it an even more vital element of her wardrobe than I did, learning a great deal from conversations with it.

DREAM IMAGES

Another way of experimenting with it is to think of the people and things as images. You can see my dialogue told me something about my image of tiger skins. There are still other possibilities for those pelts; I haven't experimented with my tiger skins meaning anything other than cloaks of power: perhaps I will one day.

Dreams sometimes play tricks or jokes on us, giving us puzzles, I sometimes think. No dream has one finite meaning. A vital dream might suggest one meaning one day, and a different one later. Someone else might have a different story to suggest about a dream. Playing with dreams and their possible images is the most flexible journal writing we can do.

Jabulani dreamt he was driving a double-decker bus along a beach – dangerous enough in itself – but driving scarily out of control from the top deck. The more he reflected upon this in his journal, the more he felt the bus was his work which was as difficult as driving on sand from the top deck. Moreover he, the bus and all the passengers might at any moment be swept into the ocean. Standing on the beach was the conductor: only he wasn't a bus conductor, he was an orchestra conductor waving his baton, conducting both the ocean waves and the bus, from the beach. And the conductor was his godfather: an old-fashioned strict army general.

Quite apart from enjoying this wonderful story as a surreal picture or film, Jabulani was able to:

1. Laugh at his work situation which had much got on top of him, affecting his sleep pattern and making him anxious. This lightening was a great relief.

2. Relocate himself from the role of top-deck driver to that of conductor on the beach (remember I said one way of playing with dreams is to think of yourself as each character or thing in the dream in turn). This helped him regain a sense of agency and authority in his role, which had been slipping. He returned to work after that journal-writing session with a straighter back and lighter step.

3. Decide the conductor's baton was perhaps a magic wand to influence his impossible work situation. He resolved to discover what the wand was an image of at work.

4. Return to the whole dream looking for different images. Perhaps the dream was about his marriage, and the conductor was his wife... But that's another story.

Jabulani has specialised in transport dreams for many years. His journal is full of bizarre accounts of cars, lorries, ships, aeroplanes, helicopters, and so on. Each one has been fruitful; had he not remembered these dreams, or not reflected upon them in writing to this depth, there is no doubt his understanding of his life would have been poorer, and he'd have been denied a dream-life richer than films.

PLAYS ON WORDS

Dreams are full of jokes and codes; images and disguised characters are not the only ones. There are also frequently puns. A pun is two words which sound the same but have different meanings and are generally spelt differently. I have a William Blake engraving print with a script: *I want! I want!* The frame is gilt; the *gilt* of the frame relates, for me, with the *guilt* involved in our culture with wanting.

One man was puzzled to dream about his feet. One time his feet stuck to a gluey floor; he was beginning to panic when he woke up shouting. Another night the skin was peeling from his feet like onions. He dialogued with his feet in his journal, asking what this was about. Still puzzled he returned to his journal after the third dream, in which the bottom of his foot had been caught by a giant crab. Rereading previous entries, he heard the words differently, and began to understand. He had repeatedly written the word *sole*. Well, apart from being Italian for sun, it is also a pun for *soul*. That made him stop and think, and write some more. Having recently passed a significant birthday and suffered several close bereavements, he hadn't been sleeping well: he realised he had got in rather a panic about dying. Luckily he was able to find the right way to talk to his wife about it, and they were able to share their grief and anxiety. He stopped dreaming his soul/sole was being torn off.

A woman dreamt she was reaching into the bag she took to work: not just her hand but the rest of her began to be sucked in, as if by a giant vacuum cleaner. Just as her head was about to disappear she woke up sweating and gasping for breath. Here's a bit of her journal:

ME: 'What were you trying to do to me, bag?'

BAG: 'I'm swallowing you up. You've got no other life, so you might as well live in me!'

ME: 'What on earth do you mean? Of course I've got plenty of life: I'm not ready to die!'

BAG: 'No not die: just become part of me for ever and ever!'

Her conversation with the bag continued, and after considerably more reflective writing the woman began to tackle how she had allowed her life to be increasingly taken over by her work. She realised she'd neglected her children, and hadn't noticed her husband was spending more and more time out. Even when at home, she was busily tapping on lap- or palm-top computer. Lucky for her she was able to make sense of the dream, realising how she was losing her life. She understood the work-bag in the dream to stand for all of her work.

PUNS, PARAPRAXES

Slips or mistakes are similar, sometimes called Freudian slips or parapraxes (I love this long word for such a simple thing). I'm including them here because of their similarity to dreams. They can be treated as if waking dreams, and subjected to similar reflective enquiry.

One man constantly mistyped *calm* as *clam* in his journal. He never noticed it, but his trusted reader did. At first he just replied, 'oh it's just a typo'. His persistent and perceptive reader insisted he reflect further. When he told himself he was being calm, he was clammed up, bottled up. He was forcing himself to appear calm: inside he was even more tense and anxious.

A man was exploring his experience of complex cancer, and noticed he'd hand-written *wife* instead of *life*. He was delighted that he felt about her in this way to this extent, and told her. It brought them even closer together.

Another man had started to see another woman. Twice he happened to leave lying around – once in a book, and then on a pile of papers – receipts from taking her out to dinner. His wife found them, but he asserted it was a mistake. When he also accidentally left lying around a love-note from the other woman, his wife made him think about it. Quite a bit of journaling later, and sharing of some of it with her, he was able to realise his anxiety: that he had possibly left the notes around for her to find and prevent him continuing the affair. Not a very responsible way of ending a relationship, and painful for the wife: but that aspect of it could be explored in his journal, shared with her, and they both tackled it together.

FAMOUS ENLIGHTENING DREAMS

Many artists rely on dreams. Paul McCartney heard the music which became *Yesterday* played in a dream by a classical string ensemble. Others look to dreams for images, characters and plots, many of them bizarre, such as the surrealist painters de Chirico, Dali, Magritte, the film director Bunuel, and the artist and writer Cocteau. Innumerable works of art owe their genesis to opium, or other drug-dream images. Cocteau wrote and drew a remarkable diary charting his recovery from opium addiction. Coleridge's popular poem *Kubla Khan* is derived from an opium-induced dream, interrupted, Coleridge said, when he was awoken by 'the man from Porlock'; he couldn't return to the dream and the poem remains incomplete.

Mary Shelley said in the 1831 preface to her novel *Frankenstein* that she had first conceived it in a dream, while staying with Lord Byron by Lake Geneva, aged eighteen (it was published when she was nineteen). The novelist Robert Louis Stevenson's *The Strange Case of Dr. Jekyll and Mr. Hyde* began with a dream. He had, from a young age, dreamed complete stories, and could go back to the same dreams on succeeding nights to give them different endings. He consciously used this skill later in life for his writing, and described dreams as 'that small theatre of the brain which we keep brightly lighted all night long' (1883). The novelist John Steinbeck said 'a problem difficult at night is resolved in the morning after the committee of sleep has worked on it' (1954, p.54). More recently Stephen King says he gleans ideas for novels such as *Misery* from dreams. In *Bag of Bones* he says, 'perhaps in dreams everyone is a novelist' (2000, p.64).

Many scientific theories begin in dreams. Srinivasa Ramanujan was a genius mathematician who learned many mathematical formulae in dreams from Hindu goddess, Namakkal.

Dreams have generally been known to be powerful, yet inscrutable. The poet Lord Byron wrote, 'Sleep hath its own world, / And a wide realm of wild reality' (1904[1816], p.146). Each person disappears into sleep and dreams, unconnected with other people: it has been likened to death. Robert Herrick in the seventeenth century wrote, 'Here we are all, by day; by night we're hurled / By dreams, each one, into a several world' ('several' means separate) (1898, p.40). Despite the cleverness of science and psychology, dreams have never been explained. Every culture has had theories as they are a large part of our experience. Australian aborigines believe dreams link them to the eternal world of *Dreamtime* ancestors. Ancient Greeks believed they had healing as well as prophetic power. Joseph earned his coat of many colours, high state position and wealth from the interpretation of dreams which foretold the future, as the Bible Old Testament tell us.

Western science has at times maintained dreams are meaningless jumbles of experience and image. Freud asserted they are the 'royal road to the unconscious' (1959, p.608), and analysed them for many patients. It has been said that Adolf Hitler, age six, was referred to Freud with terrible nightmares, but his father wouldn't hear of it, and no sessions were held.

Dreams are stories given to us by previously unknown parts of ourselves. We can invent stories which are almost as powerful. Chapter 12 talks about how to write expressive and explorative fiction.

WRITE!

1. Begin every session by writing for *six minutes* with no given subject. Allow the hand to follow the flow of whatever appears on the page: you will find subjects to write about appear on their own: if they don't, then describe something about your surroundings, or that you feel.

2. Keep a notebook by the bed.

   a. Jot notes at night to help you remember when you write more fully in the morning. Remember, a tiny dream image like a completely empty old fashioned wooden cupboard can be significant.

   b. Write the story of a recent dream in the present tense, as if it were a film, telling it in a filmic dramatic way. Include as many details as you can remember, however small or insignificant they seem.

   c. Write the dream-film title and a paragraph of blurb describing it for the cinema website.

   d. List the characters as if for a cast list (include significant objects such as 'river' as if they are characters). Write three or so words to describe each character.

   • Do any of the characters remind you of anyone (try to think widely)?

- What does the dream-film make you feel? Does it make you remember anything?

- What questions do any of the characters ask you? This might be anything!

- Write your answers.

- What question(s) would you like to ask any of them?

- Write their answers.

3. If you have ever had recurring dreams…

   a. Write what you can remember of the recurring images. For example, for years I dreamt I'd moved to a most unsuitable *huge* complicated house which was partly falling down, with none or far too little garden… Write as much as you can about the dreams.

   b. Dialogue with the characters or things, as described in Chapter 9. Ask them why you keep dreaming about them. Write their reply.

4. Reread your writing lovingly and with close uncritical attention. Amend or alter anything as it occurs to you. Add in any details which seem useful. Experiment with dialogues with characters as above, playing with any dream metaphors and puns.

Once upon a Time…

Made-up stories and poems can take a different perspective view of the self, life and work. Like writing dreams, it's another method of getting away from writing directly about the self. Yet oddly, writing about made-up characters and situations can offer significant insight into our present lives and work. Fiction can do this because it is built on personal experience: from memory, dreams, observation, dialogues, reflections and images.

WHAT IS FICTION?

Fiction opens up experimentation with what *might have happened, or could happen.* The trouble with real life is that plots come mixed up, and people do uncharacteristic and unexpected things. Writing fiction can be a way of making events and people do what your pen or keyboard make them do.

Fiction can express and explore experience. We write it from our understanding of people: the way they interact, and the way society works or doesn't work. This knowledge comes from reflection of our own experience and values, and observation of the world both directly (see Chapter 13) and through research. Plots, characters and places might be invented experiments, but what they have to say is life-like because drawn directly from life and experience.

WHERE TO START

One way is to take a real-life situation already explored in writing. It might be an event which needed the kind of reflection only writing can offer; or perhaps about a puzzling work or family event. There are many ways stories can be rewritten: substituting a happy ending for a sad, or swapping the gender of the main characters, for example. Or one can be written from the point of view, the perspective, of a main person or thing in the story other than oneself. It'll be a new story, a fiction, because you don't know what the other person really felt or knew. They become the main character, the 'I'. You become just one of the other characters. Hella wrote as from the point of view of a door she'd seen in a picture (Chapter 4). Family physician (GP) Shamini wrote as if she were the mother of a dying child patient, enabling her to perceive from her point of view (Chapter 5). Here is the beginning of a story by Heidi, a nurse and midwife, in which she writes in a patient's voice; the second paragraph discusses how it felt to write.

One of The Girls

I am fat and I fill the bed. It creaks when I move around. I hardly ever get off it, except when I waddle to the toilet and waddle back. I lie in the corner bed, by the window, far away from you. I hate you nurses. You are young and slim. You move quickly and you laugh. I am young and I was one of you. I was a nurse, and now you have to notice me. My fat is white and folds over itself between my thighs and knees. My anklebone pins my skin down. My hair is thin and I don't talk much. But I have pain and it never goes away. So I come to hospital, to you, and you give me pethidine every four hours, on the clock, all day and all night. I can make you do this to me. I can make you stupid cows see me, take notice of me, make you see and touch my skin…

For a few years I have been carrying this destructive, vengeful patient round in my head, and now having written this, have found somewhere for her to go. I was one of the smiling busy nurses that she hated so much. From her I learned that there are sometimes much deeper strong feelings which lie underneath the surface impression of people's lives and motivate their actions. These are not easily accounted for in the way that nurses and doctors like to account for things. We tend to acknowledge only the socially acceptable emotions that are comfortable to the patients, to us, and to us if we were patients. This does not include feelings such as hatred, destructiveness and a desire for chaos to be felt externally as it can be felt internally. At the time I felt this woman was, in a way, using all of us involved in her care to help her carry on a course of action which would eventually kill her.

Heidi Lyth (2003, p.100)

Writing a completely made-up fiction is an alternative. In a workshop with hospital patients we each invented a long complex journey to fetch or find something valuable: beginning by writing a phrase or several sentences in response to each of these:

1. Where are you going?

2. Why are you travelling?

3. What is your food and drink?

4. What will keep you warm at night?

5. What will protect you from dangers?

6. What do you take to remind you of home?

7. Who or what is your companion on the journey?

8. Do you have something to help you find the way?

9. Will you take something to help in case of trouble?

10. What is your most memorable form of travel?

11. What is the most dramatic bit of the journey?

12. What else do you think you need?

13. Where do you get to?

14. What do you find there?

15. How do you feel?

The resulting notes were used to create a story, writing for about 20 minutes. A woman included 'I need the compass in my head and my sense of humour… I will take with me the thought of my daughter's hug, the way my son swings me off the ground when he greets me, and the smile in my husband's eyes.' One man ended with 'I will open the door and put down my bags and say "I've arrived!"' Another: 'My destination is a place to call home. I came to fix my heartbeat.'

TALL DARK HANDSOME STRANGERS, DETECTIVES, FAIRIES, ORCS

Romantic love stories, detective stories, folk or fairy tales, fantasy, sci-fi, whodunnit, thriller are all specific forms of story. All more or less formulaic;

the writing seems less inventively demanding. For example, putting pen on the paper and writing *Once upon a time* invites a set range of characters to appear: beautiful wronged girls, wicked stepmothers, bad or good giants, talking animals, three wishes, seven brothers or dwarves, and so on. Places will also be limited to such as castles and deep dark forests. And so with situations: people will be duped, wishes will turn out differently from expected, powerful magical gifts are given, good will win out, wickedness will end up boiled in a pot.

These characters, places and situations are archetypes: they are like stock moulds found in every individual's life and work. All of us have ogres in our lives, fairy godmothers, wicked stepmothers, unattainable fairy castles and deep dark forests needing to be braved. Look at the other face of your bullying boss, and you'll see Bluebeard; that unexpected pay rise came from a fairy godmother; the new drug which worked was the gift of the magician; and so on...

Romantic fiction similarly has archetypes: she is lovely but underrated and in a minor role in life; he is strong and handsome but a bit headstrong and rich/powerful. They meet and fall inappropriately in love, difficulties occur which seem insurmountable and the relationship is broken. Someone or something dramatically intervenes and they live happily ever after.

Detective, whodunnit and thriller stories are also based on archetypes. They are often written back to front, with knowledge of the ending kept in the writer's mind so suspense can be built and readers kept guessing to the end. The whole plot works towards the denouement. It must be enormous fun to write like this, for those who can keep issues in their heads and juggle possibilities. I'd be hopeless and give the secret away immediately: I can't tell jokes, inevitably saying the punch line too early. Or these stories could just as well be written, perhaps more excitingly, with the writer waiting breathlessly until the last page to find out what happens. Part of the formula of whodunnit or detective stories are trick events or characters which put the reader off the scent.

J.R.R. Tolkein (author of *Lord of the Rings*) took the idea of writing folk tales seriously. A scholar, he realised Britain had little of its own, lost with our successive waves of foreign domination (Roman, Viking, Saxon, etc.). He set about creating a coherent mythology based on old un-destroyed texts, and drawing on mythologies from other peoples. We gained *Middle Earth* with its hobbits, dwarves, elves, wizards and other wonders and adventures.

Writing our own folk tales, or romantic fiction allows us to perceive the archetypes which have formed our lives; a constructive process. Sila wrote a fairy story which gave her life a happy ending, and punished those who hurt her. Here is the ending and her comment:

> The parents travelled back to their old village and lived quietly with their memories. Occasionally they would call for the children and then remember why they had run away. Zenus carried on with his work and Magda returned to her wine-making but sadness settled over their home, as a constant mist which would cover the sun on birthdays to remind them why their cruelty had driven their children away. Locals said the sadness was Magda's heart come back as a cloud. Only in her dreams would Magda sometimes see two young people coming towards her down their garden path. So while the children grew up happily in the castle, their parents lived their lives alone in their old house.
>
> *My writing the story was a bit like a snake shedding its skin. And it was like I wanted to remind my dad about my mum, and all that happened to us as a family, which he just seems to have forgotten, or, buried somewhere very deep. The story helped me objectify the situation. I can look at it now, and laugh at his pomposity. Even study him as an example of denial to the bitter end.*
>
> Sila Tarina

PANTOMIME AND CARTOON

Pantos, comedy and cartoons make fun of events and people considered to be serious and important. They not only relieve the tension but more seriously can enable us to take a fresh look, gaining insight thereby. Most great works have been made fun of in some way. A student wrote a sonnet: 'O my luve's like a heap of muck…' (from Robert Burns' 'O my luve's like a red red rose…'; 1993[1794], p.233). Lewis Carroll's *Alice in Wonderland* and *Through the Looking Glass* include many, such as of a Wordsworth poem. The *Mad Hatter's Tea Party* makes a comedy of Carroll's own Oxford University. Academics clearly went to sleep like the Dormouse who, on being woken, assured the meeting of Dons, 'I heard every word you Fellows were saying' (1954[1865], p.61).

Pantomimes have stock characters or archetypes (the bossy dame, the unfortunate clown who doesn't want to be funny, the hapless hero, the dim-witted but lovely girl), and in many episodes those puffed up with their own importance ultimately make fools of themselves. A senior academic of one of Britain's leading universities rewrites work experiences. Their impact is more than funny: he stands back from everyday stresses and strains and gains a wider perspective, and in laughing loses some of the strain of institutional focussing on unimportant details.

> Sixty pigs entered the boardtrough. Dark suited, grey whiskered, very few sows to hogs, they sat for three hours, as pigs were not designed to sit. Fine hoghairs were split and handed round to be sniffed and judged upon. Their achievement was to add one new criterion for *advice to examiners on when to give a first class exam result rather than a second class when the student has a borderline overall mark of 79.5%*. When the committee met again the following year they revised this important decision.
>
> *Writing this helped me know these meetings for an idiotic waste of high-powered, high-salaried academic time. I no longer contribute to the meeting as that would make it last even longer, but instead think up more ways of rewriting and poking fun.*
>
> *Stephen*

Longfellow's *Hiawatha* (see Chapter 6) has steady rhythm and a mythological narrative: ripe for making fun, as my grandfather did with this ridiculous doggerel.

> First he killed the mudjukovis
> Of its skin he made some mittens
> He to get the warmside furside inside
> turned the coldside skinside outside
> He to get the coldside skinside outside
> turned the warmside furside inside
> So he turned them insideoutside.
>
> *Tom Wignall*

PARODY

The form or the content of famous literature is often imitated, generally with a different focus from the original. It can be a rewarding way to write, as certain elements are given; everything does not have to be created from scratch.

Dracula, a brilliant Victorian romantic horror story by Bram Stoker, has been rewritten many times in writing, film, advertising and on stage. Rebecca's powerful, troubling parody is an attempt, amongst other things, to help her, as a doctor, to understand more about self-harm and obsession.

Dracula

Dracula was moonlighting as a phlebotomist. He reflected on the irony of this as he ventured out into the daylight. He had been so lonely and now he had a chance to make new friends. He had a thick accent, which repulsed people. He wasn't very popular with the few other Transylvanian exiles he had met since his arrival. They thought him strange and difficult. They didn't realise that his somewhat brusque manner was more to do with his physical discomfort than any desire on his part to rebuff them. The light was a problem. His skin chafed and burned and he broke out in a dreadful rash. He had trouble with his eyes. So he went to his GP, who prescribed a steroid skin cream and some eye drops.

Everything went well at first. He was skilled at taking blood, and the sight of it made him feel warm inside. But then things began to go wrong…

Rebecca Ship (2001, p.73)

In the final full chapter we reflect more upon the nature of personal *Key* writing, what elements it is made up of, its foundations.

WRITE!

1. Begin every session by writing for *six minutes* with no given subject. Allow the hand to follow the flow of whatever appears on the page: you will find subjects to write about appear on their own: if they don't, then describe something about your surroundings, or that you feel.

2. Fiction: Here are some suggested headings. Include as many details as come to your mind. If none of these works for you: try again another time, or alter my list to suit you better.

   • Describe an empty room. It is one where something has been happening, and something further is going to happen.

   • Someone enters the room; who are they, what's their name, why are they there and what do they do?

   • Another person enters. Who? Do they know each other already? What do they think of each other? What happens between them?

   • A creature (animal/insect/fish/magical being…) comes into the story: in what way?

   • Some event or disaster occurs, or they have an argument.

   Make up the rest…

3. Write the story of your life, or a chapter from it, as one of these or similar.

   a. How might it start?

   • It might be a romantic love story: a lovely girl stuck in a difficult situation, ready to be rescued…?

   • Or a whodunnit: the detective calmly enjoying life and then hearing of the murder…?

   • Perhaps a fantasy: a fantastic situation of space ship or strange land and oddly named beings…?

   • A fairy or folk tale: Once upon a time…?

   • Or an adventure story: a mundane peaceful perhaps boring situation, and then…?

   b. Put the first sentence on the page and allow your pen or pencil to follow the flow of your mind. Don't worry about what is going to happen; just begin at the beginning and allow the story to write itself. Or, especially if it's a whodunnit, begin mapping the plot as if it were a comic strip, like a storyboard.

c. Write or plan for as long as you can without stopping to think. Allow yourself to live the story as your hand writes.

4. Write about an event in your life (anything; it might not seem significant when you start) in as much detail as you can. Now:

    a. write again about that event from the point of view of someone else who was there; or

    b. write another piece, changing the ending or another aspect of it to make it even happier or more significant in some way; or

    c. try rewriting it, swapping the gender of one or more character, perhaps yourself (if you are male tell the story as if you are female); or

    d. even set it in another time in history, or in another culture, or alter it in some other significant way: be imaginative!

5. Write a story making fun of a situation or a piece of writing you know well. Or an irritating event in your life, or one that made you angry, or wryly amused. You can turn family members or colleagues into whatever you like, as Lewis Carroll turned Oxford dons into a Mad Hatter, a March Hare and a Dormouse (you need never show it to them). Start writing in a similar way as for 3.

6. Read your writing, including the *Six Minute Write*, to yourself and make any alterations to the content which seem appropriate. And remember you have five senses.

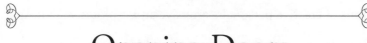

CHAPTER 13

Opening Doors

Key writing can open doors to sunshine and light. This chapter suggests the underlying fundamental questions it grapples with, and explains how they can be explored through the four basic methods of creative personal expressive and explorative writing.

FOUNDATIONS OF *KEY* WRITING

Fundamental questions addressed by writing are:

- Who are you?

- What is important in your life and world?

- Which people are vital to your life?

- Where do you come from, and where might you be going?

- When did significant events happen for you?

- How does your life cohere, fit together, and how can you now make the best of it?

- WHY? WHY? WHY? (Children and scientists are never quite satisfied with answers, nor should we be.)

Responding to these can enable us to see ourselves, our world, and society and culture as if through new glasses. These questions can be responded to on many levels: practically, factually, logically, emotionally, spiritually, imaginatively. They can be thought of in terms of me, my work, family, home and personal environment, or about political, cultural, sociological, theological, historical ideas theories and so on. We each determine our own focus.

These questions can be explored in four different ways, the four foundations of creative personal expressive and explorative writing:

1. *Observation and description* of anything such as the natural and constructed world, people, work, society, events.

2. *Reflection* on anything inside, such as feelings, memories, dreams, thoughts, aspirations, fears, ambitions.

3. *Metaphor creation*: putting things together which aren't associated in real life. In Chapter 1, expressive writing was likened to keys unlocking doors to rooms and walled gardens. This is a metaphor because it's not literally about locks, keys and doors. Our language is shot through with metaphors, so much we rarely notice (see Chapter 7).

4. *Narration* of an event (e.g. the birth of our first baby, that successful experiment). Telling or narrating stories about our lives comes naturally, and can help make sense of experience. Writing narratives increases their reflective power. Written stories draw on reflection, observation and image.

All personal writing draws upon some or all of these four ways of writing. Poetry makes particular use of them all. Observation and reflection are like lock and key. Image experimentation is like penetrating oil slipping in to ease and dissolve mental stiffness. Turning a key in a well-oiled lock gives intrinsic pleasure in a well-working mechanism. Narration is like the handle to turn and push the door open. Story offers the continuity of plot with beginning, middle and end, encouraging development of ideas and inspirations; plots gain their own dynamic, carrying the writing forward. Fiction, building on the stable power of narrative, can take writers into new dimensions. Sometimes these fresh dimensions can be surprising and illuminative, just as playing with images can be.

The four foundations dance with each other. Reflection underpins image and story; many stories are image-laden; all stories include acute observation; and so on. In my journal I recently described cherry blossom: observation. This led to thinking and rereading about ancient formal Japanese observation writing. Cherry blossom is an essential Japanese image for both the fragility and power of human life. Although the blossom only lasts a few days, it comes back every year, just as new babies are born and fresh life-chances happen. This flower image writing led me, via thinking about the vase of dying white lilies on my desk, to some deep reflection concerning my mother. I wrote a fictionalised story about her death.

Another example. Writing which reflects upon specific dreams (e.g. what the dream was about, who and what was in it, what you felt) leads swiftly to image exploration. Jabulani dreamt he was riding a motor bike through thick mud; gradually it changed to a toy motor bike which got smaller and smaller, and then the handlebars fell off. Reflecting upon the dream led him to relate it to a request he'd given much thought to the previous day to give a prestigious lecture. He had considered saying yes, because he had much experience to share. The dream, and writing about it afterwards, led him vehemently to realise he really didn't want to do it; that he'd retired from academic life and had written his wisdom in books these people could read, and going backwards to give the lecture would be like riding a toy bike with no handlebars in thick mud. He wanted to look forward to his new life; mostly playing his new (very old but refurbished) grand piano.

Balance between observation, reflection, image and story generally happens naturally. It can be unpredictable and surprising, though. Generally no-one can plan to be creative at any one time or place, nor how they will be creative. *Writers' block* is the down-side. When I trust this writing, have respect for myself doing it, and am willing to give myself the gift of time, space and energy in doing it, then my own balance occurs naturally. My *Key* writing is fruitful and enjoyable, though never systematic or predictable. This mini-story incorporates an observation which enabled and supported reflection.

> My learning of how to be with my father on his last day came from the exemplary care given by a young nurse as she fed him at mid-day. From my journal: 'She feeds him a few spoonfuls of semolina. She looks lovingly into his eyes, calling him by his first name. His eyes open wide. I am taken by surprise at this contact of the young nurse feeding him, and then washing his mouth with such love and care. He is very responsive and alert.'

> I feel privileged to have had that time with him. If I had not watched that young nurse who allowed herself to show love for her patient, a dying

man, a stranger, then I don't think I would have quite known how to show love towards my own father, and had such an intense experience.

Monica Suswin

The balance between observation, reflection, image creation and narration can occasionally get out of kilter. A strategy for when stuck and dissatisfied with writing is to reread it, and try some based on a foundation which seems to have been lacking recently. Getting stuck on observation writing can lead to feeling it's not getting anywhere and is boring. Too rich a diet of reflection can feel too self-centred and introverted. Too much metaphor and simile can lead to lack of contact with everyday life, a kind of dislocation. Over-indulgence in fiction or story can begin to feel insufficiently located in explorative imaginative work. Here is the beginning of a real life story:

'I can't cope with life – I'm too different'

At 8.58am June 4 2001, the staff at Gloucestershire Royal Hospital Accident Unit surrendered and pronounced my son dead. He was twenty-two. He had been brought in by the police who had gone to pick him up after a householder had reported him behaving strangely. As the policemen approached him he stuffed the plastic bags he had retrieved from bins into his mouth and choked. Those bags contained dog excrement.

Revolting? Yes. To be condemned? No. Not if you knew the story behind what this young man did.

Robbie was born after a mismanaged labour. He was yanked into the world by misapplied forceps which damaged nerves linking his brain to his body. He could not suck, he could not swallow his own secretions. He was termed a 'floppy baby' and after multiple tests was assumed brain damaged. We, his parents, were told that it was unlikely that he would ever walk or talk. I did not believe them – his eyes told me otherwise. The medical profession talked tests, weights and tube-feeding. I talked love, touch, home. I discharged him without medical consent. I'd learnt how to tube-feed him, aspirate him, do everything they did for him in the special needs unit. Robbie started to show signs of wanting to live…

My rough draft was a powerful emotional experience – I just let it pour out, and with it my grief and my memories. It was a cathartic and healing thing to do. My re-writing and editing of it forced me to be more objective and in

so doing allowed me to feel more 'whole'. I wrote a series of poems at the time,
which came to chart my grieving process from just before Robbie's death to
about a year later. That was my release.

Judy Clinton (2004, p.50)

Writing is a release, and so very much more as Judy discovered as she
worked on and redrafted, and also used reflective strategies to deepen her
appreciation and extend her understanding of her work. *The Writer's Key:
Creative Solutions for Life* has explored a large arena of possibilities. Now,
with the very last chapter, you, my reader, begin to take the keys fully into
your own hands.

WRITE!

1. Begin every session by writing for *six minutes* with no given subject.
   Allow the hand to follow the flow of whatever appears on the page:
   you will find subjects to write about appear on their own: if they don't,
   then describe something about your surroundings, or that you feel.

2. Observation: write lists of things you notice today, observing with all
   your senses. Invent your own list headings, or use these:

   - things from the natural world

   - things from the built environment

   - something about a person or people

   - items from the news or other media

   - an element from a work or home habitual activity, such as typing
     an email, cooking…

   Each might be one word or a phrase, or each might become a paragraph
   or so. You might find you write much more about one element, and not
   continue the list. That's great: return to the rest another time (having
   started once more with the *Six Minute Write*). My poem, *Charney
   Manor*, written from daily observations, is in Chapter 3.

3. Reflection: continue writing from the sentence stems below; see
   where they take you. Do one in great detail, or do them all with only
   a sentence: allow whatever comes. It's the sort of thing you could

do many times, and write something different each time (though just occasionally nothing comes).

- When I…
- The door opened…
- Where might we…
- If only…
- Who could help…
- What if…

4. Narration: write a story of:

- a Christmas memory
- a birthday memory
- a holiday memory
- an event you know happened but can't remember
- a surprise
- an animal in your life.

5. Metaphors.

a. Make a quick dashed list of words about something important to you, your work, hobby, child, a favourite place. Words might be *stressful, sympathetic, stimulating.*

b. Choose a positive word to begin with (*stimulating* rather than *stressful*); write it at the top of a page.

What pictures does this word bring into your mind? Remember, even if some of them seem odd, they will all be right.

- Stimulating is a talk with Sam.
- Stimulating is a cup of coffee just at the right time.
- Stimulating is, when I've got sleepy at a meeting, going outside into the wind for a couple of minutes.
- Stimulating is a shower of rain in a hot day.

c. Reread your list when you begin to run short of ideas. Reorder them and think about relationships between items. This might give further ideas.

6. Reread all your writing including the *Six Minute Write*. Make any changes that occur to you which develop your thinking or understanding, or make the writing come more alive. Write notes on your reflections on rereading. Show the writing to a trusted confidential other, asking for their opinion and advice, if you think it would help.

CHAPTER 14

Ever After

I love the way the writing process is not solely an act of will. Much of it is subterranean, sometimes choosing unexpected words to wake us from sleepwalking or to explain our experience to ourselves. Even writing's silences, the fallow periods, have their reasons. If we respect its ways, writing can be a life-long companion, patient enough to hold our hand through every year's changes.

Robert Hamberger (2008, p.126)

River found writing helped her as a young person struggling through personal difficulties:

Death opened the door and shoved a pen and paper in my hand. I was a reluctant writer, an unlikely poet. In 1986, when I was 22, my mother was diagnosed with ovarian cancer. Through sheer despair I started to write, first in journals, later in poems.

My journals of the time record vivid dreams and vicious encounters with jealousy and insecurity. It was deeply exciting to move the pen across the page, to be given permission to write from experience.

River Wolton (2008, p.126)

Yang found a route to dealing with the impossibility of having far too much to do in her life. A computer systems engineer, she worked at full stretch when there, and then came home to a busy family life. Her previous strategy had been to create a timed programme for each day; her problem was that the tight timetable always slipped, making life more and more stressful.

Yang discovered she had assumed she was responsible for far too much. She did this by working through *The Writer's Key* strategies, including lists, the most useful of which was entitled: 'Things I don't have to do!' To her amazement this list got longer and longer as she realised some self-imposed tasks were just unnecessary, and others she'd delegated to someone else. Her second most useful list was 'Things I've noticed today', which had to include things from nature, about her colleagues and family members, things she smelt, touched and tasted as well as saw. The narrow box of her life widened to include thrush-song heard while walking to her car each morning, and that the formerly unnoticed habitual flower arrangement in her office foyer was not only fabulously coloured, but scented. One day she was startled to be offered promotion. She couldn't know if it had any relationship to the life changes her writing brought; but she did wonder if expanding her creativity so enjoyably and absorbingly, and taking more control over her life, had a wider impact on her future than she could have imagined.

THE WAY FORWARD

Continue to write. *The Writer's Key* has given the main ideas about unlocking your life through writing. All these methods can be built upon, such as different ways of writing unsent letters, dialogues, stories and poems, and viewing dreams.

Joining a writing group can take writing into a new arena. Many groups are a wonderful support and help; they can be found through social media, the internet, at local libraries or community colleges, or adverts in local shops, post offices or newspapers. If the first one doesn't seem right, try another: they are enormously different.

Writing can help find out what we think, know, feel, experience, remember and understand. It is an ally when making difficult life decisions, clarifying an argument, understanding someone else's point of view. Life so often seems ambiguous and complex. Writing can enable exploration of what we think about specific issues (personal, work, political, social, spiritual), life values, as well as what we need and want.

You don't need a book to tell you what to do next with your writing, my reader. You don't need to ask: 'what do you think I should do with my writing, this or this?' If you asked me I'd reply: 'I don't know, ask your writing!' Recently I said this in response to an email, and the person replied within seconds: 'oh thank you: I know what to do now.' 'Don't thank me', I think: 'thank yourself'. The key is in your hand, put it in the lock, turn it and open the door to find a whole creative world beyond: simply by writing.

APPENDIX A

TYPES OF EXERCISES AND ACTIVITIES

Writer's Key exercises are listed below according to type. The areas of life they can help with is then given, followed by the chapters to find them in.

Autobiography/reminiscence

Self-confidence and racial identity	C5
To leave record for future generations	C5
Understand self better	C1, 2, 3, 5
Understanding life's trajectory better	C5

Blogging

Birthright HIV	C3
Stillbirth	C3
Terminal illness	C3

Doodles and diagrams

How to use	C3

Dialogue

Life clarity (dreams)	C11
Life traumas and experiences	C9, 10

Dreams

Enlightenment: from typos, etc. (parapraxes)	C11
How to write from and about	C11
Retirement	C13
Significant life issues	C11
Terminal illness	C1
Work–life balance	C11

Fiction

Personal/professional development	C12, 13

Good conditions/materials for writing

Bereavement	C2
Bullying at work	C3
How to find	C1, 2, 3, 6

Pictures
Bereavement C4
Unhappy childhood C4

Place
Life clarification C4, 11
Post traumatic stress disorder C4

Poetry
Depression C1, 6
How to write C6
Significant life experiences C6
Work–life balance C6

Point of view, seeing from another
Personal development C6
Professional development C3, 5, 8, 11

Reflective journal writing
Failed job interview C3
Fear of flying C1
Professional reflection C3, 5, 6, 11
Serious illness C1, 3

Sentence stems, developing writing starting from
General (list of sentence stems) C1, 3, 5, 13
Severe illness (I wish…) C1

Sharing writing with appropriate other
How to C2

Six Minute Writing
Dynamic job change C2
How to… C2
Personal and professional development C3
Substance abuse C2

Things
Disturbed remembrance of childhood C4
Disturbed remembrance of relative C4
General (clothes) C3
How to write poetry C6
Life clarification (found objects) C4
Life clarification (significant objects in life) C4

Tin openers (how, why, what, who, when, where)

    Clarity (checklist)   C3, C13

    How to write poetry   C6

    Reflect upon significant events   C2

Titles for writing

    Various headings   C4, 5, 13

Trance writing

    To bring peace and mindfulness   C3

Sent letters

    Enabling communication   C8

Story writing

    How to write   C12

    Personal understanding (through genre)   C12

    Professional understanding (through genre)   C12

    Reflect on significant professional events   C5, 12

    Reflect on personal events   C5, 12, 13

Unsent letter writing

    Life traumas and experiences   C8, 9, 10

EXERCISES AND ACTIVITIES TO HELP WITH SPECIFIC AREAS

Writer's Key exercises are listed below according to the areas of life they can help with. The type of exercise is then given, followed by the chapters to find them in.

Issues, specific

Starting big project	Metaphor and image	C3
Gaining peace of mind	Observation	C3, 13
	Dialogue	C10
	Lists	C4, 6, 13, 14
	Trance writing	C3
Decision making	Lists	C3
Understanding others	People, observation	C4, 11
	Point of view	C3, 5, 6, 8, 9, 11
Communication	Sent letters	C8
Record for future	Reminiscence	C5
Reminiscence	People	C4
	Story	C1, 2, 3, 5, 15
	Things	C4
Success	Dialogue	C10
Parenting	Dialogue	C10

Personal development

	Clothes	C3
	Dialogue	C9, 10, 11
	Dreams	C11
	Fiction	C12
	Internal mentor	C8, 9
	Internal terrorist	C9
	Lists	C10
	Metaphor and image	C8, 10, 11, 13
	Objects	C4, 6
	People	C4
	Place	C4, 11
	Reflective journal writing	C6
	Sentence stems	C1, 3, 5, 13

	Story writing	C5, 12, 13
	Tin openers	C2, 3, 6, 13
	Typos and parapraxes	C11
	Unsent letters	C8, 9, 10

Problems, specific

Substance abuse	Dialogue	C9
	Six minute writing	C2
	Letter writing	C8
Bereavement	Dialogue	C9
	Pictures	C4
	Unsent letters	C8
	Writing in the right place	C2
HIV (child)	Blogging	C3
Stillbirth	Blogging	C3
Racial identity	Autobiography	C5
Unhappy childhood	Pictures	C4
Relationship problems	Metaphor and image	C8
Phobia	Metaphor and image	C8
	Reflective journal writing	C1
Lack of confidence	Keywords	C3, 5
	Poetry	C10
PTSD	Place	C4
	Metaphor and image	Preface
Stress/depression	Dialogue	C9
	Reflective journal writing	C1
	Poetry	C6
	Place	C4
Neighbour difficulty	Metaphor and image	C8
Being replacement child	Poetry	C5
Phantom limb	Unsent letters	C8
Anger/guilt	Unsent letters	C8
	Sent letters	C8
Physical illness	Unsent letters	C8
Mental illness	Unsent letters	C8
Reflecting on work	Fictionalised life stories	C3, 5, 6, 11, 12, 13
	Genre story writing	C12
	Lists	C14
	Materials for writing, etc.	C3
	Metaphor and image	C8
	Point of view	C3, 5, 6, 8, 11
	Six minute writing	C3
	Story writing	C5

REFERENCES

Abse, D. (1998) 'More than a green placebo.' *The Lancet 351*, 9099, 362–4.

Barrett Browning, E. (1993) 'How do I love thee? Let me count the ways.' In *The Oxford Library of English Poetry*. Oxford: BCA.

Blake, W. (1970[1794]) *Songs of Innocence and Experience*. London: Oxford University Press.

Burns, R. (1993[1794]) 'A Red Red Rose.' In *The Oxford Library of English Poetry*. Oxford: BCA.

Byron, Lord G. (1904[1816]) 'The Dream.' In *Byron Complete Poetical Works* (ed. F. Page). Oxford: Oxford University Press.

Carroll, L. (1954[1865]) *Alice's Adventures in Wonderland*. London: J.M. Dent and Sons.

Clinton, J. (2004) 'I can't cope with life, I'm too different.' In 'Opening the Word Hoard' (ed. G. Bolton). *The Journal of Medical Ethics: Medical Humanities 30*, 1, 50-51.

Coleridge, S.T. (1970[1834]) *The Rime of the Ancient Mariner*. London: Dover.

Frank, A. (1947) *The Diary of Anne Frank*. London: Macmillan Children's Books.

Freud, S. (1959) *The Standard Edition of the Complete Works of Sigmund Freud*, Vol. V. London: Hogarth.

Hamberger, R. (2008) 'Saying My Name.' In *Hand Luggage Only* (ed. C. Whitby). Leicestershire: Open Poetry.

Hamilton, F. (2012) 'Writing in a changing world.' *Lapidus Journal 6*, 2, 12–14.

Helfgott, E.A. (2012) 'Diary of my husband's illness: after his death – still witnessing Alzheimer's.' *Journal of Poetry Therapy 25*, 1, 39–48.

Herrick, R. (1898) *The Hersperides and Noble Numbers*, Vol. 1 (ed. A. Pollard). London: Lawrence and Bullen.

Homer (1996) *The Odyssey* (trans. R. Fagles). New York, NY: Penguin Viking.

Hopkins, G.M. (1953) *Poems and Prose* (ed. W.H. Gardner). London: Penguin.

Hughes, T. (1982) 'Foreword.' In S. Brownjohn, *What Rhymes with Secret?* London: Hodder and Stoughton.

Jenkinson, S. (2003) 'The unequal struggle.' In 'Opening the Word Hoard' (ed. G. Bolton). *The Journal of Medical Ethics: Medical Humanities 29*, 1, 51–2.

Keillor, G. (1985) *Lake Woebegone Days*. New York, NY: Viking Penguin.

King, S. (2000) *On Writing: A Memoir of the Craft*. New York, NY: Simon and Schuster.

Kipling, R. (1902) *Just So Stories*. London: Macmillan.

Knight, J. (2012) 'These are the Stories Doctors Tell.' In M. Hulse and D. Singer (eds) *The Hippocrates Prize Anthology of Winning and Commended Poems*. London: Hippocrates Press.

Latham, J. (2006) 'Man on Street Corner...'; 'Not to be Measured by its Length'. In *Sailor Boy*. Wales: The Collective.

Longfellow, H.W. (1960[1854]) *The Song of Hiawatha*. London: J.M. Dent and Sons.

Lyth, H. (2003) 'One of the girls.' In 'Opening the World Hoard' (ed. G. Bolton). *The Journal of Medical Ethics: Medical Humanities 29*, 2, 100.

Michelson, J. (2005) 'Letting in the light, a work of therapeutic art' (ed. G. Bolton). *Progress in Palliative Care 13*, 2, 68–71.

Morrison, B. (1993) *And When Did You Last See Your Father?* London: Granta Books.

Nesbitt, E. (1996/1997) 'Writing cancer out of your life.' *Link Up 46*, 7–9.

Nimmo, D. (1993) 'Kill the Black Parrot.' In *Kill the Black Parrot*. Todmorden: Littlewood Arc.

Petrone, M.A. (2002) 'The tattooed intruder.' In 'Opening the Word Hoard' (ed. G. Bolton). *The Journal of Medical Ethics: Medical Humanities 28*, 1, 29–30.

Praxilla (1996) *Classical Women Poets* (trans. and intro. J. Balmer). Tarset: Bloodaxe Books.

Proulx, A. (1993) *The Shipping News*. London: Fourth Estate.

Rhys, E. (2002) 'Lost in France: Jo's Requiem.' In M. Taylor (ed.) *Lads: Love Poetry of the Trenches*. London: Gerald Duckworth.

Rich, A. (2006) Acceptance speech for the National Book Awards medal for distinguished contribution to American Letters. Available at www.nationalbook.org/nbaacceptspeech_arich. html, accessed 22 May 2013.

Sappho (1996) *Classical Women Poets* (trans. and intro. J. Balmer). Tarset: Bloodaxe Books.

Shonagan, S. (1967) *The Pillow Book of Sei Shonagan* (trans. and ed. I. Morris). London: Penguin.

Ship, R. (2001) 'Dracula.' In 'Opening the Word Hoard' (ed. G. Bolton). *The Journal of Medical Ethics: Medical Humanities 27*, 2, 72–3.

Starkey, H. (2004) 'Warts.' In 'Opening the Word Hoard' (ed. G. Bolton). *The Journal of Medical Ethics: Medical Humanities 30*, 2, 93.

Steinbeck, J. (1954) *Sweet Thursday*. London: Penguin.

Stevenson, R.L. (1883) *Across the Plains*. Available at http://classiclit.about.com/library/bl-etexts/ rlstevenson/bl-rlst-acr-1.htm, accessed on 30 August 2013.

Stubbersfield, A. (2006) 'Dying of the Light.' In *Joking Apart*. Wales: The Collective.

Tennyson, A. (2007[1851]) 'The Eagle.' In *Selected Poems: Tennyson* (Penguin Classics). London: Penguin.

Tennyson, A. (1993) 'The Lady of Shallott.' In *The Oxford Library of English Poetry* (ed. J. Wain). Oxford: Oxford University Press.

Wilde, J. (2003) 'Vietnam on Saturday. Monday in Limavady.' In S. Denyer, L. Boydell and U. Hearne (eds) *Reflecting Leadership. Dublin and Belfast: Institute of Public Health in Ireland*.

Winterson, J. (2011) *Why Be Happy When You Could Be Normal?* London: Jonathan Cape.

Wolton, R. (2008) 'Death and Poetry: How Writing Helps Us Say the Unsayable.' In G. Bolton (ed.) *Dying, Bereavement and the Healing Arts*. London: Jessica Kingsley Publishers.

Woods, C. (2008) 'First Thing.' In *Dangerous Driving*. Manchester: Comma Press.

Woolf, V. (1979[1931]) 'Professions for women.' In *Virginia Woolf: Women and Writing*. (ed. and intro. M. Barrett). London: The Women's Press.

Wordsworth, W. (1976) 'Preface.' In *Lyrical Ballads* (ed. D. Roper). Plymouth: Macdonald and Evans.

Yeats, W.B. (1903) 'Adam's Curse.' In *In the Seven Woods*. London: Macmillan.